T0362533

Hot Topics in Cosmetic Dermatology

Editor

HASSAN I. GALADARI

DERMATOLOGIC CLINICS

www.derm.theclinics.com

Consulting Editor
BRUCE H. THIERS

January 2024 • Volume 42 • Number 1

ELSEVIER

1600 John F. Kennedy Boulevard ● Suite 1800 ● Philadelphia, Pennsylvania, 19103-2899

http://www.theclinics.com

DERMATOLOGIC CLINICS Volume 42, Number 1
January 2024 ISSN 0733-8635, ISBN-13: 978-0-443-18390-4

Editor: Stacy Eastman
Developmental Editor: Nitesh Barthwal

Dermatologic Clinics (ISSN 0733-8635) is published quarterly by Elsevier Inc., 360 Park Avenue South, New York, NY 10010-1710. Months of publication are January, April, July, and October. Business and editorial offices: 1600 John F. Kennedy Blvd., Suite 1800, Philadelphia, PA 19103-2899. Customer service office: 11830 Westline Drive, St. Louis, MO 63146. Periodicals postage paid at New York, NY, and additional mailing offices. Subscription prices are USD 447.00 per year for US individuals, USD 478.00 per year for Canadian individuals, USD 547.00 per year for international individuals, USD 100.00 per year for US students/residents, USD 100.00 per year for Canadian students/residents, and USD 240 per year for international students/residents. For institutional access pricing please contact Customer Service via the contact information below. International air speed delivery is included in all *Clinics* subscription prices. All prices are subject to change without notice. **POSTMASTER:** Send address changes to *Dermatologic Clinics*, Elsevier Health Sciences Division, Subscription Customer Service, 3251 Riverport Lane, Maryland Heights, MO 63043. **Customer Service: 1-800-654-2452 (U.S. and Canada); 314-447-8871 (outside U.S. and Canada). Fax: 314-447-8029. E-mail: journalscustomerservice-usa@elsevier.com (for print support); journalsonlinesupport-usa@elsevier.com (for online support).**

Reprints. For copies of 100 or more, of articles in this publication, please contact the Commercial Reprints Department, Elsevier Inc., 360 Park Avenue South, New York, New York 10010-1710. Tel.: 212-633-3874; Fax: 212-633-3820; Email: reprints@elsevier.com.

The *Dermatologic Clinics* is covered in *MEDLINE/PubMed (Index Medicus), Current Contents/Clinical Medicine, Excerpta Medica, Chemical Abstracts,* and *ISI/BIOMED.*

Contributors

CONSULTING EDITOR

BRUCE H. THIERS, MD
Professor and Chairman Emeritus, Department
of Dermatology and Dermatologic Surgery,
Medical University of South Carolina,
Charleston, South Carolina, USA

EDITOR

HASSAN I. GALADARI, MD, FAAD
Associate Professor of Dermatology,
Department of Internal Medicine, College of
Medicine and Health Sciences, United Arab
Emirates University, Al Ain, United Arab
Emirates

AUTHORS

JANA AL-HAGE, MD
Dermatologist and Venereologist, Department
of Dermatology, Saint Louis Hospital, AP-HP,
Groupe Hospitalier, Paris, France

LEENA AMIRI, MD
Assistant Professor, Department of Psychiatry
and Behavioural Sciences, College of Medicine
and Health Sciences, United Arab Emirates
University, Al Ain, United Arab Emirates

RICHARD ROX ANDERSON, MD
Director, Department of Dermatology, Harvard
Medical School, Wellman Center for
Photomedicine, Massachusetts General
Hospital, Boston, Massachusetts, USA

MATHEW AVRAM, MD, JD
Dermatologist, Department of Dermatology,
Harvard Medical School, Wellman Center for
Photomedicine, Massachusetts General
Hospital, Boston, Massachusetts, USA

MAHSA BABAEI, MD
Post-Doc Research Fellow, School of
Medicine, Stanford University, Stanford,
California, USA

FOTINI BAGEORGEOU, MD
Dermatologist and Venereologist, Chemical
Peeling Department, Andreas Sygros Hospital
of Dermatological and Venereal Diseases,
University Clinic, National and Kapodistrian
University, Athens, Greece

LUIGI BENNARDO, MD
Dermatologist and PhD candidate, Department
of Health Sciences, Magna Graecia University,
Catanzaro, Italy

FRANCESCO P. BERNARDINI, MD
Oculoplastic Surgeon, Oculoplastica
Bernardini, Genova, Italy

VINCE BERTUCCI, MD, FRCPC, FAAD
Dermatologist, Department of Medicine,
University of Toronto, Toronto, Ontario,
Canada; Private Practice, Woodbridge,
Ontario, Canada

ANDRE BRAZ, MD
Dermatologist, Private Clinic, Rio de Janeiro,
Brazil

RISHI CHOPRA, MD
Laser & Cosmetics Expert, Department of
Dermatology, Harvard Medical School,
Wellman Center for Photomedicine,
Massachusetts General Hospital, Boston,
Massachusetts, USA

KINNOR DAS, MD
Consultant Dermatologist, Apollo Clinic,
Silchar, Assam, India

ALIA GALADARI, MD
Dermatologist and Venereologist, Saint Louis
Hospital, APHP, Paris, France

HASSAN I. GALADARI, MD, FAAD
Associate Professor of Dermatology,
Department of Internal Medicine, College of
Medicine and Health Sciences, United Arab
Emirates University, Al Ain, United Arab
Emirates

MICHAEL H. GOLD, MD
Dermatologist, Gold Skin Care Center,
Tennessee Clinical Research Center, Nashville,
Tennessee, USA

MOHAMAD GOLDUST, MD
Post-Doc Research Fellow, Department of
Dermatology, Yale School of Medicine, New
Haven, Connecticut, USA

STEFANIA GUIDA, MD, PhD
Assistant Professor, Dermatology, Vita-Salute
San Raffaele University, Milano, Italy

WILSON W.S. HO, MBChB, FRCSEd
The Specialists: Lasers, Aesthetic and Plastic
Surgery, Hong Kong

CHRISTINA HUANG, MD
Dermatologist, Department of Dermatology,
University of Toronto, Toronto, Ontario,
Canada

OMAR A. IBRAHIMI, MD, PhD
Wellman Center for Photomedicine,
Massachusetts General Hospital, Boston,
Massachusetts, USA; Founding and Medical
Director, Connecticut Skin Institute, Stamford,
Connecticut, USA

MARIA CLAUDIA ISSA, MD, PhD
Professor of Dermatology, Department of
Internal Medicine, Fluminense Federal
Fluminense, Rio de Janeiro, Brazil

SYED FAHAD JAVAID, MD
Assistant Professor, Department of Psychiatry
and Behavioural Sciences, College of Medicine
and Health Sciences, United Arab Emirates
University, Al Ain, United Arab Emirates

MARTIN KASSIR, MD
Dermatologist, Worldwide Laser Institute,
Dallas, Texas, USA

SALONI KATOCH, MD
Consultant Dermatologist, Dr. KN Barua
Institute of Dermatological Sciences,
Guwahati, Assam, India

SAMAR KHALIL, MD
Dermatologist, Skin & Scalpel Clinic, Sin el Fil,
Lebanon

SUZANNE KILMER, MD
Dermatologist, Wellman Center for
Photomedicine, Massachusetts General
Hospital, Boston, Massachusetts USA; Laser &
Skin Surgery Center of Northern California,
Sacramento, California, USA

EVGENIYA ALTAROVNA KOGAN, MD
Department of Anatomic Pathology, Sechenov
University, Moscow, Russian Federation

A.YU. KOROLEVA, MD
Center for the Treatment of Complications of
Professor Yutskovskaya's Clinic, Moscow,
Russian Federation

MARINA LANDAU, MD
Dermatologist, Department of Plastic and
Reconstructive Surgery, Shamir Medical
Center, Be'er Ya'aqov, Merkaz, Israel

SHIR BLUM LANDAU
Co-Founder, MAHUT Ltd, Herzliya, Israel

TINGSONG LIM, MD
Clique Clinic, Kuala Lumpur, Malaysia

STEVEN PAUL NISTICÒ, MD, PhD
Professor, Head of Department of
Dermatology, Department of Health Sciences,
Magna Graecia University, Catanzaro, Italy

ELIANDRE PALERMO, MD
Dermatologist, Private Clinic, Sao Paulo, Brazil

ASHAKI D. PATEL, MD
Dermatologist, Department of Dermatology,
Harvard Medical School, Wellman Center for

Photomedicine, Massachusetts General
Hospital, Boston, Massachusetts, USA

GYANESH RATHORE, MD
Dermatologist, Department of Dermatology,
Military Hospital, Dimapur, Nagaland, India

FERNANDA H. SAKAMOTO, MD, PhD
Assistant Professor, Department of
Dermatology, Harvard Medical School,
Wellman Center for Photomedicine,
Massachusetts General Hospital, Boston,
Massachusetts, USA

RASHMI SARKAR, MD, FAMS
Director Professor, Department of
Dermatology, Lady Hardinge Medical College,
SSK and KSC Hospital, New Delhi, India

ELISABETTA SCALI, MD, PhD
Department of Health Sciences, Magna
Graecia University, Catanzaro, Italy

BRENT SKIPPEN, MD
Oculoplastic Surgeon and Ophthalmologist,
Wagga Wagga, New South Wales, Australia;
UNSW Medical School, Sydney NSW, Australia

MARTINA TOLONE, MD
Dermatologist, Department of Health
Sciences, Magna Graecia University,
Catanzaro, Italy

INES VERNER, MD
Dermatologist,Verner Clinic for Dermatology
and Aesthetics, Tel Aviv, Israel

YA.A. YUTSKOVSKAYA, MD
Cosmetologist and Dermatovenerologist,
Dermatovenerology and Cosmetology
Department, Pacific State Medical University of
Health, Moscow, Russian Federation

ELENA ZAPPIA, MD
Department of Health Sciences,
Magna Graecia University, Catanzaro,
Italy

Contents

Cosmetic procedures involve the maintenance, restoration, or enhancement of one's physical appearance through surgical or medical techniques. Restorative or reconstructive procedures, on the other hand, are essential procedures that restore normal function or appearance to abnormal structures caused by trauma or infection. Cosmetic procedures are generally elective and may either be surgical or nonsurgical. Nonsurgical or minimally invasive cosmetic procedures include laser hair or tattoo removal, chemical peeling, micro-dermabrasion, and soft tissue augmentation with injectables. These procedures are fast-growing with more than a 50% increase globally over the last 5 years.

Skin specialists and practitioners are commonly requested to recommend on cosmetic products to improve skin appearance and address certain "non-medical" concerns. During residency and further education, dermatologists rarely expand their knowledge regarding cosmetic ingredients, except if they are a cause of medical condition or disease, such as contact dermatitis. This review provides guidelines to the INCI list structure, together with basic principles of cosmetic products formulation.

Chemical peeling is a procedure used for cosmetic improvement of the skin or treatment of some medical skin disorders, by the application of chemical exfoliant. In spite of a long history of clinical use of chemical peels, understanding of the science behind the procedure is still evolving. In this article, we review new concepts, understandings, and publications in the field of chemical peels.

Superficial chemical peels are one of the most popular skin resurfacing procedures in a dermatologists' clinic today due to quick application process, fast recovery, good patient acceptance, and excellent cosmetic results. The role of various peeling agents like glycolic acid, salicylic acid, trichloroacetic acid, Jessner's solution, retinoic acid, and lactic acid in the management of melasma has been established as that of an additional or maintenance therapy. This article details the current evidence and recommendations for the use of chemical peels in the treatment of melasma, a chronic and recurrent hyperpigmentary disorder.

material when filling large zones. An in-depth understanding of the facial anatomy and ongoing training are crucial for practitioners to develop and improve technical abilities.

Lower eyelid skin is unique and different from that of other areas. In addition to being an area of high exposure to the sun and elements, there are anatomic considerations and specific histologic characteristics that can cause the skin in this area to be more sensitive. These attributes can readily cause under-eye wrinkling and pigmentation. This review aims to present an updated overview of the current knowledge regarding the clinical characteristics, diagnosis, and management of wrinkles and pigmentation in this area. These disorders are usually caused by different factors, such as genetics, aging, sun exposure, lack of sleep, and stress.

Knowledge of the anatomy of the infraorbital region is key to understanding the full extent of clinically visible infraorbital defects and the underlying structures involved to achieve optimal aesthetic results. The authors have developed a more anatomic approach to the infraorbital region, which has led to recognition of a specific anatomic area, defined previously as the aesthetic G-point. Shifting attention away from the tear trough itself and applying a surgical approach to aesthetic medicine can lead to more natural and complete results while at the same time minimizing the risk of undesired side effects and complications.

 Video content accompanies this article at http://www.derm.theclinics.com.

Cosmetic surgeons have conventionally used the line of ligaments to guide facial lifting or volumizing procedures. However, this line is only partially reliable in determining the limits of the mobile and fixed face, as the low point of this line was described in front of the movable jowl fat. This article proposes a new understanding of the ligament. To address this concept, the authors entitled this line the functional ligament line. This article links facial anatomy and its changes during movements to the injectable fillers according to their mechanism of action and rheologic properties.

Hyaluronic acid and calcium hydroxylapatite (CaHA) have been used for in the field of soft tissue augmentation. Both materials have been used in combination to enhance tissue remodeling and provide a more rejuvenated look. Sequential injections of Belotero Volume (CPM-HA V) and CaHA had a relatively greater remodeling effect on one's skin compared with the simultaneous injections of CPM-HA V and CaHA.

DERMATOLOGIC CLINICS

SERIES OF RELATED INTEREST

Medical Clinics
https://www.medical.theclinics.com/
Immunology and Allergy Clinics
https://www.immunology.theclinics.com/
Clinics in Plastic Surgery
https://www.plasticsurgery.theclinics.com/
Otolaryngologic Clinics
https://www.oto.theclinics.com/

DERMATOLOGIC CLINICS

THE CLINICS ARE AVAILABLE ONLINE!
Access your subscription at:
www.theclinics.com

Preface
Cosmetic Experiences from Across the Globe

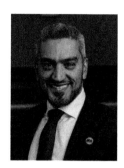

Hassan I. Galadari, MD, FAAD
Editor

The pursuit of beauty is as old as humanity itself. Over the centuries, cultures around the world have developed diverse beauty rituals and skincare techniques, each reflecting their unique values and traditions. The world of cosmetic dermatology has been expanding exponentially. This expansion was helped by the intricate ability of the world to connect. The ease by which practitioners from across the globe can share their knowledge and experiences in a scientific medium, through publications as well as congress presentations, has been paramount in making cosmetic procedures safe and accessible. In this issue of *Dermatologic Clinics*, care has been taken to cover basic aspects of cosmetic dermatology in an updated form as well as shed some light on new innovations in the pipeline. Whether you are a seasoned dermatologist seeking to expand your knowledge or an inquisitive reader with an interest in the science of beauty, this comprehensive guide aims not only to enlighten and inspirebut also to be practical in its approach to help translate that knowledge into everyday clinical practice.

As the demand for cosmetic procedures continues to rise, it is essential to strike a balance between artistry and safety. Topics that highlight the perception of beauty, clinical assessment to the delivery of procedures have been made into focus and the avoidance of certain practices that may lead to unfavorable outcomes are highlighted.

What truly stands out, however, is that care has been taken to include global leaders from different parts of the world. This inclusivity helps in creating the microcosm of what is now a reality: that knowledge and experience are but a click away. It is our intention that this issue will serve as an invaluable resource for professionals in the field, empowering them to provide the highest standard of care.

While many specialties have recently put claim on the field of cosmetic dermatology, the understanding of skin, its disease condition, and management, whether therapeutic or cosmetic in nature, ultimately falls on the shoulders of the dermatologist.

Hassan I. Galadari, MD, FAAD
College of Medicine and Health Sciences
United Arab Emirates University
PO Box 15551
Al Ain, UAE

E-mail address:
hgaladari@uaeu.ac.ae

Dermatol Clin 42 (2024) xiii
https://doi.org/10.1016/j.det.2023.08.006
0733-8635/24/© 2023 Published by Elsevier Inc.

The Effects of Cosmetic Procedures on the Youth

Leena Amiri, MD[a], Syed Fahad Javaid, MD[a], Alia Galadari, MD[b], Hassan I. Galadari, MD[c],*

KEYWORDS

• Youth • Cosmetic procedures • Body image

KEY POINTS

• The increased demand for cosmetic procedures is a current issue among the youth between 18 and 34 years of age.
• Cosmetic procedures in the youth carry potential risks, including complications related to anesthesia, infection, scarring, unrealistic expectations, psychosocial impact, and long-term effects.
• It is important for young people to fully understand these risks and to have appropriate support and counseling throughout the process.

INTRODUCTION

Cosmetic procedures involve the maintenance, restoration, or enhancement of one's physical appearance through surgical or medical techniques.[1] Restorative or reconstructive procedures, on the other hand, are essential procedures that restore normal function or appearance to abnormal structures caused by trauma or infection.[2] Cosmetic procedures are generally elective and may either be surgical or nonsurgical.[1] Nonsurgical or minimally invasive cosmetic procedures include laser hair or tattoo removal, chemical peeling, micro-dermabrasion, and soft tissue augmentation with injectables.[3] These procedures are fast-growing with more than a 50% increase globally over the last five years.[4] Such a global surge in demand can be partly attributed to the effects of social media and exposure of certain patient population groups to what these procedures are.[4]

The increased demand for cosmetic procedures is a current issue among the population between 18 and 34 years of age.[5] The reasons of why this population group is drawn toward such procedures are yet to be fully explored, but may include

amplified body concerns, a matter seen in the changing bodies of adolescents.[5] While cosmetic procedures are becoming increasingly popular among youth, the decision to undergo any such procedure should not be taken lightly. It comes with its own set of benefits and risks. Factors influencing the decision to undergo such procedures include societal pressures, body image issues, and self-esteem.[6] There is a lack of well-designed studies and standardized nomenclature of cosmetic procedures for nonmedical reasons.[5,6] There is also an imbalance of publications internationally, mainly in the non-Western population.[5] This review article provides a breakdown of the effects of cosmetic procedures on youth and provides several recommendations, including improving evidence-based nonmedical reasons for undergoing cosmetic procedures.

DEFINING YOUTH

Youth generally refers to the period between childhood and adulthood, which can vary depending on cultural, social, and economic factors.[7] This period is characterized by physical, psychological, and social changes.[7] In general, youth is associated

ª Department of Psychiatry and Behavioural Sciences, College of Medicine & Health Sciences, United Arab Emirates University, PO Box 15551, Al Ain, United Arab Emirates; ᵇ Saint Louis Hospital, APHP, 1 Avenue Claude Vellefaux, Paris 75010, France; ᶜ Department of Internal Medicine, College of Medicine & Health Sciences, United Arab Emirates University, Al Ain, United Arab Emirates
* Corresponding author.
E-mail address: hgaladari@uaeu.ac.ae

https://doi.org/10.1016/j.det.2023.06.009
0733-8635/24/© 2023 Elsevier Inc. All rights reserved.

with a period of transition, where individuals start to develop their own identities, form relationships, and make important life choices.[7] It is a time of both mental and physical growth with unique challenges and opportunities.[7]

FACTS AND NUMBERS WORLDWIDE

Cosmetic procedures among youth are on the rise.[8] According to the American Society of Plastic Surgeons (ASAPS), the number of cosmetic procedures performed on patients aged 19 years or younger in the United States alone was nearly 240,000 in 2018,.[9] Of these procedures, botulinum toxin injections have increased by 28% among patients aged 18-24 years old between 2010 and 2018.[9] Furthermore, a survey conducted by the American Academy of Facial Plastic and Reconstructive Surgery (AAFPRS) found that 64% of members reported an increase in cosmetic surgery or injectable treatments in patients under age 30.[9]

Although there are no updated statistics in the United Kingdom, according to the British Association of Aesthetic Plastic Surgeones (BAAPS) there has been an increasing trend of cosmetic procedures.[9] Globally, South Korea has the highest rate of cosmetic procedures among young adults, with approximately 40% undergoing a cosmetic procedure during their twenties.[10] One study revealed that 8 out of 10 women in South Korea above 18 years of age stated their need to undergo a cosmetic procedure.[10] In China, numerous college students opt for cosmetic procedures to enhance their job acceptance rates, and in Singapore, there has been a 30% increase in cosmetic procedure rates, recorded between 2005 and 2010, among individuals younger than 21 years.[11]

BODY IMAGE AND THE PURSUIT OF BEAUTY

Body image is defined as the mental image of an individual's own body that is shaped by perceptions, emotions, and physical sensations.[12] The "real self," which is the actual or objective self, is processed via self-image. Self-image is subjective, while the ideal self is achieved by self-actualisation. Charles Horton Cooley has coined the "looking-glass" theory, which is divided into three parts:[12]

1. Our imagination of how we must appear to others in social situations.
2. Our imagination and reaction to what we feel their judgment of appearance must be.

3. Our development of our sense of self and responding through perceived judgments of others.

Personal identity and self-perception are formed early in life.[5] An individual's perception of attractiveness is guided by innate preferences such as symmetry and small waist-to-hip ratio amongst women.[3] Furthermore, self-esteem is the extent to which an individual values and accepts themselves.[3,12] Self-esteem, in addition to cognitive performance and mental health, may be affected by the individual's surroundings.[3,12,13] Experiencing bullying or teasing can cause lower levels of physical attractiveness, leading to an increased risk of psychological distress. As such, poor psychological functioning and a greater desire for cosmetic procedures may entail.[14,15]

Cosmetic procedures are usually driven by the desire to increase self-confidence and thinking favorably of one's self, or their desire to fit in. Therefore, the greater the psychological investment in physical appearance and internalization of mass media messages of beauty, the more favorable the attitude toward cosmetic procedures.[13]

DISSATISFACTION WITH APPEARANCE

Puberty is a time of rapid changes in the body and a time when many young individuals feel the pressure to fit in with their peers.[8] This pressure, combined with issues such as body shaming, can lead to dissatisfaction with one's appearance and a desire to seek cosmetic procedures.[14] Negative emotions such as low self-esteem, anxiety, and depression are also linked to dissatisfaction with appearance and peer pressure.[14]

Cosmetic procedures are seen as a way to improve appearance and self-esteem but may only offer temporary solutions.[9] It is, therefore, necessary for young people to seek support and counseling to address any underlying psychological issues.[11] They must also consider the potential risks and benefits of any cosmetic procedure and have realistic expectations.

SCREENING FOR BODY DYSMORPHIC DISORDERS

It is estimated that 7-15% of individuals seeking cosmetic procedures have body dysmorphic disorders (BDD).[16,17] BDD is defined as the preoccupation with an imagined or minimal defect in appearance according to the Diagnostic and Statistical Manual of Mental Disorders, 5th Edition (DSM 5).[12,16] If not screened prior to undergoing a cosmetic procedure, this might lead to paradoxically significant negative outcomes, such as high levels of psychopathology and low self-esteem.[14] Early recognition of symptoms and referral for appropriate care can help avoid such negative outcomes.[14]

Healthcare professionals should take a comprehensive approach when evaluating young people considering cosmetic procedures, including assessing physical and mental health and exploring any underlying psychological factors contributing to dissatisfaction with appearance.[10,13] They play a crucial role in promoting positive self-image and self-confidence in young.[18]. Strategies such as therapy, education, and support around healthy lifestyle habits and positive self-talk can promote positive body image and self-esteem.[9,13]

MAIN FACTORS DRIVING INDIVIDUALS TOWARD COSMETIC PROCEDURES

The concept of eternal youth and beauty is a general aspiration that has been documented since early years of civilization. In ancient Egypt, emphasis on physical appearance was made evident by the creation of perfumes, oils, and other beauty treatments.[2,11] In ancient Greece, individuals deemed most beautiful were revered.[2] The quest of finding "La Bella Figura" starts with the individual's body image and attitude toward their physical appearance.[1,2]

1- Sociocultural trends

The way we perceive beauty is shaped by sociocultural standards, as stated by the sociocultural theory. People learn about beauty standards within their cultural context, and these standards have a significant influence on individual preferences[3]. The human body is a subject of change that can affect social connections, cultural norms, beliefs, and values, with dominant social standards centering on cultural norms.[5] For instance, the extent to which cosmetic procedures are accepted plays a role in people's attitudes toward them.[9] While hearing about other individuals' experiences with cosmetic procedures may enhance interest, discrepancies in social attitudes are observed across different geographies and ethnicities, with women being more affected than men.[9]

Sociocultural trends are fuelling the rise in demand for cosmetic procedures among youth, particularly due to society's emphasis on physical appearance.[19] Youth feel pressured to conform to societal beauty standards, with social media platforms providing a space for individuals to showcase their appearance and receive feedback from peers.[11,13] Additionally, cosmetic procedures have become more socially acceptable and accessible, with many marketed toward younger individuals.[5,6]

It is important to note that not all youth seeking cosmetic procedures do so solely due to societal pressures or low self-esteem. Many have valid reasons, such as addressing medical conditions or injuries, improving physical function, or aligning their appearance with personal values and goals.[2,6] While sociocultural trends contribute to the demand for cosmetic procedures among youth, individuals should carefully consider their motivations and consult with a qualified medical professional before making any decisions. It is important to understand that the decision to undergo a cosmetic procedure is a personal one, and it's essential to ensure that one is doing it for the right reasons and is aware of the potential benefits and risks.[2,10] Ultimately, youth should be encouraged to embrace their natural beauty and unique qualities while making informed decisions about their appearance.[13,14,19]

2- Peer pressure in cosmetic procedures in youth

Peer pressure, particularly through social media, can influence young people's decisions to undergo cosmetic procedures. Impressionable youth may be challenged to undergo a certain procedure by their peers to be accepted amongst them. Parents and educators must promote positive body image and self-esteem.[12,13] The decision to undergo a cosmetic procedure should be made with careful consideration of risks, benefits, and personal goals, with the guidance of a qualified medical professional.[10,13]

3- The role of media

Traditional media formats such as television, newspapers, adverts, and online media, especially social networking sites, carry a presumed influence on seeking cosmetic procedures. Information regarding cosmetic procedures, such as before and after photographs, practice information, and online competitions, are shared on various online social media platforms. Media, therefore, can influence social ideals in body image and the "ideal body" type one should have. Generally, there is a positive endorsement of media highlighting the importance of females pursuing beauty ideals.[12,14]

GENDER VARIATIONS

The prevalence of cosmetic procedures is higher among women, with approximately 90% of procedures performed on women, despite the growing number of men opting for such procedures in the United States and the United Kingdom.[14] Women are more interpersonally oriented and thus may be more concerned about socialization experiences, which can explain why they tend to objectify their bodies with increased body surveillance habits.[14] However, gender variations and sexual orientations also play a role in undergoing cosmetic procedures. Differences in the types of procedures sought by males and females have been observed in various studies. For instance, according to the American Society of Plastic Surgeons, females aged 13-19 were more likely to seek breast augmentation. In contrast, males in the same age group were more likely to seek gynecomastia surgery.[9] Similarly, a survey conducted by the online website "Real Self" in 2020 found that females under 35 were more likely than males to research breast augmentation, while males were more likely than females to research gynecomastia surgery.[20] However, it's important to note that these are just a few examples, and the reasons for seeking cosmetic procedures can vary widely between individuals, regardless of gender.[21]

ASSESSMENT AND COUNSELING

Procedural counseling and psychological assessment are paramount to provide both reassurance and accurate information. Medical professionals must have a good conversation regarding risk-benefit and an open dialogue to fully assess the young individual's motivation and ensure realistic expectations.[9,13] Physical, emotional, psychological, social, ethical, and legal aspects all need to be detailed and unfolded. This should be followed by a 3-month cooling period if no medical justification is found, and another consultation in the presence of a parent or guardian, if consented by the capacitous patient.[10,13] Allowing more time between preliminary visit, information procedure, and ultimate procedure consent can help estimate if the wish for undergoing a cosmetic procedure persists.[10]

Reverting to the ethical issue at hand, principles of proportionality need to be asserted, and the evaluation of cosmetic procedure appropriateness based on possible risks and benefits is essential.[9,10] Generally, three main aspects need to be understood, including the psychosocial condition of the adolescent, functionality of organ(s) of interest, as well as the expected vs realistic outcomes.[10] Procedure outcomes include risks, poor results, side effects & social issues.[9]

TYPES OF COSMETIC PROCEDURES

The age range for cosmetic procedures can vary based on individual needs and health, with some guidelines as follows[3,5,8].

- Facelift surgery has no specific age limit if the person is in good health.
- Breast augmentation is most frequently done on women aged 20-35 but can still be considered for those over 35 if physically healthy.
- Liposuction is commonly performed on individuals aged 18-35 with good physical shape and skin elasticity.
- Rhinoplasty is typically performed on individuals over 18 but is more common in those aged 25-35.
- Botulinum toxin treatments are popular among individuals aged 20-35 as a preventative measure or for early signs of aging but are more commonly performed for those over 35.

It is important to consult with a qualified doctor to determine the best cosmetic procedure options based on individual needs and health.[19]

POSSIBLE BENEFITS OF COSMETIC PROCEDURES

Cosmetic procedures in youth can provide a wide range of benefits.[9,10,21] These benefits include improved self-confidence and self-esteem, which can have a positive impact on mental health and overall well-being. In addition, some procedures can address physical abnormalities, such as cleft palate repair or correction of a deviated septum, which can improve quality of life by addressing issues that may affect social, academic, or professional opportunities.[6,8] Medical benefits can also be achieved through cosmetic procedures, such as improving breathing or reducing discomfort caused by excess skin or fat.[14] Immediate physical benefits such as higher energy levels, increased activity, or reduced pain have been reported in the general adult population.[10,18] However, no empirical studies on long-term benefits have been reported in the youth.[4] It is important for young people to carefully consider the potential risks and ethical considerations associated with cosmetic procedures, and to have realistic expectations.[12] Before undergoing any cosmetic procedure, young people should fully understand the potential risks and benefits.[19]

POSSIBLE RISKS OF COSMETIC PROCEDURES AND POSTPROCEDURAL COMPLICATIONS

According to the literature, adolescent patients mostly had safer procedures with lower complication rates after undergoing face, breast, and body procedures compared to adults.[5,6,14] The most common postoperative complications in adolescent patients were hematoma (0.34%) and infection (0.28%). However, a risk-benefit ratio is a key clinical requirement to establish the appropriateness of cosmetic procedures.[5] In addition, many cosmetic procedures require the use of anesthesia, which can carry risks such as allergic reactions or respiratory problems.[5,9] In young people with developing immune systems, any surgical procedure carries a risk of infection and scarring.[5]

Psychological risks include the possibility of influencing well-being for worse.[21] A possible identity crisis may arise in adolescents of Asian background (ie, Chinese, Korean, or Philippine) after undergoing blepharoplasty to "broaden the eyes" to obtain a westernized look. Other psychological risks include lowered self-esteem and increased risk of anxiety. Depression, worsening of body dysmorphic disorders, as well as social isolation might ensue.[14] It is important for young people to have a realistic understanding of what cosmetic procedures can and cannot achieve.[11,14] They should also have appropriate support and counseling throughout the process to help manage their expectations and cope with any psychosocial impact the procedure may have.[14] Studies are lacking in understanding how cosmetic procedures influence mental health changes in youth.

FUTURE OF COSMETIC PROCEDURES IN YOUTH

As society becomes more accepting of cosmetic procedures, it is possible that more young people will choose to undergo such procedures. Additionally, advancements in technology and medicine may improve the safety and effectiveness of these procedures, making them more attractive to young people.[5,19] However, it is important to consider the potential risks and ethical concerns surrounding cosmetic procedures in youth. Therefore, there may be increased regulations or guidelines in place in the future to ensure that these procedures are performed safely and ethically.[12] There may also be a shift toward more natural and noninvasive cosmetic treatments, which could appeal to young people concerned about the risks and complications of surgery.[8] Ultimately, the future of cosmetic procedures in youth will depend on a variety of factors, including societal attitudes, medical advancements, and regulatory considerations.[14,21]

SUMMARY

As the number of cosmetic procedures among youth increases globally, it is important to consider the benefits and risks of such procedures, especially for young patients. While cosmetic procedures may boost a young person's confidence, weighing the psychological and physical risks involved is essential. Parents, healthcare professionals, and regulatory bodies should work together to guide and support young patients considering cosmetic procedures.

Professionals should manage patients on a case-by-case basis. They should be made aware of the medical, ethical, legal, and sociocultural issues in addition to all the inner motivational factors pertinent to everyone's personality and psychology. Furthermore, clinical knowledge gaps should be addressed as well as using quantifiable scales and questionnaires pre and postcosmetic procedures. This provides reliable data on their efficacy, helps understand the reasons for such procedure-seeking behavior, provides reliable information on care experiences, and improves future decision-making.

CLINICS CARE POINTS

Medical professionals performing cosmetic procedures are expected to implement the following[2,5,9,14,19].

- Play an important role in anatomy education and appreciating normal variations and physiological changes, with special attention given to adolescents.
- Obtain a complete medical, sexual, and gynecological history to ensure the absence of sexual or psychological dysfunction, including body dysmorphic disorders.
- Discuss the possibility of unintended consequences of cosmetic procedures on various areas of the body and the lack of high-quality evidence regarding outcomes.

DISCLOSURE

None.

REFERENCES

1. Swami V, Chamorro-Premuzic T, Bridges S, et al. Acceptance of cosmetic surgery: personality and individual difference predictors. Body Image 2009; 6(1):7–13.

2.. Bouhadana G, Aljerian A, Thibaudeau S. The reconstruction of plastic surgery: a historical perspective on the etymology of plastic and reconstructive surgery. Plastic Surgery 2021;1:1–5.

3. Rohrich RJ, Cho MJ. When is teenage plastic surgery versus cosmetic surgery okay? Reality versus hype: a systematic review. Plast Reconstr Surg 2018;142(3):293e–302e.

4. Markey CN, Markey PM. Emerging adults' responses to a media presentation of idealized female beauty: An examination of cosmetic surgery in reality television. Psychology of Popular Media Culture 2012;1(4):209.

5. Khunger N, Pant H. Cosmetic procedures in adolescents: what's safe and what can wait. Indian Journal of Paediatric Dermatology 2021;22(1):12–20.

6. Souad M, Ramdane T, Ghada T, et al. Cosmetic surgery and body image in adolescents: a psycho-sociological analysis of the causes and effects. Int J Humanit Soc Sci 2018;8(10):129–35.

7. Youth (1985) United Nations. United Nations. Available at: https://www.un.org/en/global-issues/youth.

8. Amiri L, Galadari H, Al Mugaddam F, et al. Perception of Cosmetic Procedures among Middle Eastern Youth. The Journal of Clinical and Aesthetic Dermatology 2021;14(12):E74.

9. Alotaibi AS. Demographic and cultural differences in the acceptance and pursuit of cosmetic surgery: a systematic literature review. Plastic and Reconstructive Surgery Global Open 2021;9(3).

10. Seo YA, Chung HIC, Kim YA. Experience and acceptance of cosmetic procedures among South Korean women in their 20s. Aesthetic Plast Surg 2019;43:531–8.

11. Wen N. Celebrity influence and young people's attitudes toward cosmetic surgery in Singapore: the role of parasocial relationships and identification. Int J Commun 2017;11:19.

12. Hermans AM, Boerman SC, Veldhuis J. Follow, filter, filler? Social media usage and cosmetic procedure intention, acceptance, and normalization among young adults. Body Image 2022;43:440–9.

13. Wen N, Chia SC, Xiaoming H. Does gender matter? Testing the influence of presumed media influence on young people's attitudes toward cosmetic surgery. Sex Roles 2017;76:436–47.

14. Lee K, Guy A, Dale J, et al. Adolescent desire for cosmetic surgery: associations with bullying and psychological functioning. Plast Reconstr Surg 2017;139(5):1109–18.

15. von Soest T, Kvalem IL, Wichstrøm L. Predictors of cosmetic surgery and its effects on psychological factors and mental health: a population-based follow-up study among Norwegian females. Psychol Med 2012;42(3):617–26.

16. American Psychiatric Association. Diagnostic and statistical manual of mental disorders: DSM-5. 5th edn. Washington, D.C: American Psychiatric Publishing; 2013.

17. Ashikali EM, Dittmar H, Ayers S. Adolescent girls' views on cosmetic surgery: a focus group study. J Health Psychol 2016;21(1):112–21.

18. AlShamlan NA, AlOmar RS, Al-Sahow AZ, et al. Cosmetic surgeries and procedures among youth in Saudi Arabia: a cross-sectional study of undergraduate university students in the Eastern Province. Postgrad Med 2022;98(1160):434–40.

19. Wood PL. Cosmetic genital surgery in children and adolescents. Best Pract Res Clin Obstet Gynaecol 2018;48:137–46.

20.. Őry F, Láng A, Meskó N. Acceptance of cosmetic surgery in adolescents: the effects of caregiver eating messages and objectified body consciousness. Curr Psychol 2023;42:15838–46.

21. Walker CE, Krumhuber EG, Dayan S, et al. Effects of social media use on desire for cosmetic surgery among young women. Curr Psychol 2021;40:3355–64.

Hacking the International Nomenclature of Cosmetic Ingredients List- How to Read Ingredients in Cosmetic Products and What Is Important for a Dermatologist to Know?

Marina Landau, MD[a],*, Shir Blum Landau[b]

KEYWORDS

• INCI • Cosmetic ingredients • Actives • Emollients • Humectants • Fragrance • Preservatives

KEY POINTS

- Dermatologists are the most likely professionals to recommend a cosmetic product to improve skin appearance or to eliminate contact with a specific cosmetic ingredient in case of allergic reaction.
- To do so, dermatologists need to be able to decipher the list of cosmetic ingredients as they appear in INCI list on the product.
- INCI list contains internationally recognized systematic names to identify cosmtic ingredients4. Basic understanding of how to read the INCI list is required from every skiun specialist.

During the past decades, medicine has expanded its limits from disease treatment to disease prevention, from providing medications to supporting health and well-being. This evolution had a significant effect on skin specialists and practitioners, who are commonly requested to address aging of allegedly healthy skin and provide advice on skin maintenance and beauty. As such, skin specialists are the most likely professionals to recommend a cosmetic product to improve skin appearance and address certain "non-medical" concerns.

During residency and further education, dermatologists rarely expand their knowledge regarding cosmetic ingredients, except if they are a cause of medical condition or disease, such as contact dermatitis.

According to the current regulation, accepted in most of the countries, all cosmetic ingredients must be labeled on the skin care or cosmetic product packaging for the user's knowledge and safety. In most cases, it is a long list with multiple chemical and botanic terms, hardly familiar to anybody.

And yet, skin specialists should possess a certain level of knowledge to be able to decipher this exhausting list of ingredients, their patients' skin is exposed to. The ability to spot the exact ingredient can be of the superior importance in case of allergic sensitivity. Even if existing in minimal amounts, the allergen can induce skin rash, which persists as long as the exposure continues.[1] Evidently, patients allergic to certain ingredients of cosmetics should be supplied with the INCI names of their allergens. Therefore, dermatologists should be familiar with INCI names.[2]

A cosmetic ingredient is any substance or raw material used to make a cosmetic product, such as skincare, hair care, makeup, or personal care

[a] Department of Plastic and Reconstructive Surgery, Shamir Medical Center, Be'er Ya'aqov, Merkaz, Israel;
[b] MAHUT Ltd, Herzliya, Israel
* Corresponding author. 2 Hashunit street, Herzliya, Israel
E-mail address: dr.marinaclinic@gmail.com

Dermatol Clin 42 (2024) 7–11
https://doi.org/10.1016/j.det.2023.06.006
0733-8635/24/© 2023 Elsevier Inc. All rights reserved.

items. They can be derived from natural sources, such as plants, minerals, or animals, or they can be artificially produced. According to the international regulation standards, and similarly to the food industry, it is mandatory for all the ingredients in a cosmetic product, to be labeled on the product container or package. This list of ingredients is called INCI list, or International Nomenclature of Cosmetic Ingredients list. INCI list contains systematic names, internationally recognized to identify cosmetic ingredients. The INCI system was established in early 1970's and is maintained by the International Cooperation on Cosmetics Regulation (ICCR), which is an organization seeking to harmonize the regulation of cosmetics in different countries, including USA, Brazil, Canada, China, Taipei, EU, Israel, Japan, Korea, and so forth (https://www.iccr-cosmetics.org/). Any person, institution or company, which developed, found or isolated a new compound and want it to be registered and listed in INCI, can apply with supporting materials. Listing of an ingredient in INCI list, does not mean that the ingredient has been approved for cosmetics or assessed for safety or efficacy. Assessment of the cosmetic ingredients is performed by Cosmetic Ingredient Review independently.

WHY IS INTERNATIONAL NOMENCLATURE OF COSMETIC INGREDIENTS LIST NEEDED?
Name of the Ingredient

Some cosmetic ingredients possess multiple names - chemical, common, trade name, and so forth. A standardized non-commercial name is assumed to make our lives easier and allow a decent comparison between cosmetic formulations. The truth is, that most INCI names are nonintuitive and are very different from their commonly used names and are a mixture of conventional scientific names, Latin and English words. This makes the INCI list challenging to navigate. For example- INCI name for water is aqua. Vitamin C is listed in INCI as L-Ascorbic Acid (**Table 1**).

The list of INCI names can be found in the Glossary of Common Ingredient Names published by the European Commission. INCI names can also be accessed via the Cosmetic Ingredient database (https://ec.europa.eu/growth/tools-databases-cosing.index.cfm?fuseaction=searc. simple), found online on the European Commission website for cosmetics.

Order of the Ingredient

Each manufacturer/brand has a "secret recipe" for a cosmetic product, so there is no possibility to find the exact concentration of each ingredient in the

Table 1 Example of the commonly used names versus the respective INCI names	
Commonly Used Name	**INCI Name**
Aloe vera	Aloe barbadensis
Tea tree oil	Melaleuca alternifolia
Lavender oil	Lavandula angustifolia
Balsam of Peru	Myroxylon Pereiare
Parabens	Benzylparaben, butylparaben, ethylparaben, methylparaben, propylparaben
Kathon CG	Methylisothiazolinone, methylchloroisothiazolinone
Amerchol L101	lanolin alcohol and paraffinum liquidum

formulation. Generally, the ingredients appear in an order reflecting their concentration: the ingredients at the top of the list are those with highest concentration in the formula, and from there down, the ingredients are listed in a descending concentration order. If the raw material is supplied as a mixture, each individual ingredient is declared separately, considering its concentration in the finished product.

According to most of the regulations, ingredients which concentration is lower than 1% do not have to appear in a particular order in the list. There are some hints that can be concluded from the product label. For example, certain ingredients have a maximal approved concentration. Therefore, one can assume what is a concentration of the ingredients preceding or following them.

Plants, Colors, Scents, Allergens, and Nanomaterials

In Europe the plants are named by the generally accepted nomenclature of Linnnaeus, which is a rank-based scientific classification of organisms (for example Aloe barbadensis is aloe vera), while in the USA botanic ingredients are labeled by their common names (eg, Rosmarinus Officinalis (rosemary) extract).

In Europe the dyes, other than dyes used to color hair, appear at the end of the list without a specific order by means of Color index (CI) Number. For example, blue No.1 will appear as CI420290. In the US Color additives are named according to the FDA Color additive name (eg, FD&C Yellow No. 5). For perfume and aromatic compositions in Europe, the INCI names "parfum" or "aroma" is used, while in the USA perfumes and flavors are listed as "fragrance" and "flavor". While FDA does not require to declare the presence of known allergens, in Europe presence of any of the 26 allergens listed in Annex III of the Cosmetics Regulation 1223/2009 has to be specifically declared in the ingredients list, if their concentration exceeds 0.001% for leave-on products (eg, face cream) or 0.01% for rinse-off products (eg, shower gel). In case a product contains nanomaterials, this has to be clearly indicated by using the word "nano" in brackets next to INCI name of the nanomaterial (eg, titanium dioxide [nano]). In the USA the trade secret ingredients may be listed at the end of the ingredient list, using the phrase "and other ingredients."

Function of the Ingredients

But what do those long names in the ingredient list mean and what do they do? While the formula of each product may differ, most cosmetics contain a combination of at least some of the following core ingredients: excipients, additives and actives. The excipient is a base on which the product is developed. It can be a cream, a lotion, a gel, an emulsion, a foam. The most common excipients are water, glycerin, alcohol, silicones. Additives are products incorporated into skincare products to provide more pleasant appearance and better preservation. They are usually responsible to the products smell, color and specific texture: softness, stickiness, and so forth. Actives are important for the specific product's activity: antiaging, bleaching, and so forth. As in medications, the activity of the ingredients also depends on its concentration. Unlike with medications, in skincare products the exact concentration of the actives is not labeled, therefore the presence of a specific active ingredient does not reflect its activity (eg, presence of 0.1% ALA in cosmetic products). Therefore, product with a very long list of allegedly active ingredients is not necessarily a better product.

ACTIVES (OR FUNCTIONAL INGREDIENTS)

The variety of active substances is wide and their presence in the formula depends on its purpose.

- In firming formulas, components such as retinol or its natural derivative Bakuchiol are used to promote the natural production of collagen.[3–5]
- Antiaging activity of the skin care is one of the most socially desirable effects.[6] Active ingredients promoting proliferation and differentiation of keratinocytes supporting regulation of epidermal protection barrier against mechanical and chemical insults.

- In anti-pigmentation products components such as alpha-arbutin or Niacinamide are included.[7–10]
- Products designed for oily, or acne prone skin include ingredients such as salicylic acid, or its natural derivative – white willow bark extract[11,12]
- For anti-antioxidant skin protection, vitamin C, or its botanic derivatives (such as camu camu and others) are added.[13–15]
- Restoration of the epidermal barrier function is one of the uppermost important functions of skin care products. With better understanding of the molecular mechanisms involved in the differentiation and function of the epidermis, many cosmetic products target this aspect for a better looking and healthier skin.[16] Ceramides restore the intercellular structure of the epidermal barrier, while urea can substitute for natural moisturizing factor (NMF).[17–19]

EMOLLIENTS AND HUMECTANTS

Water is essential for the normal functioning of the skin and especially its outer layer, the stratum corneum. Natural retention of water in the stratum corneum is dependent on 2 major components: (1) the presence of natural hygroscopic agents within the corneocytes (collectively referred to as natural moisturizing factor) and (2) the stratum corneum intercellular lipids orderly arranged to form a barrier to transepidermal water loss.[20]

To moisturize the skin artificially by using cosmetic products, a "water retainer" and "evaporation protector" are needed. "Water retainers" or hydrators are called humectants. Evaporation protectors are emollients or occlusives. An emollient and a humectant are not the same nor they are built to serve the same purpose.

The relative proportion of emollients and humectants differ in different skin care products. Emollient-enriched preparations are especially important in patients suffering of atopic dermatitis, hand eczema, age-related xerosis, and so forth. Highly oily emollients may also serve as occlusive agents, by coating the skin with a thin oily film that seals the water inside, thus keeping the skin hydrated for longer.

A recent TikTok trend called *Slugging* refers to exactly that. Beauty influencers apply a petroleum-based product over their usual moisturizer or serum and leave it on overnight to increase the occlusive effect on the skin to reduce transepidermal water loss and increase water retention. On the other hand, these preparations (or TikTok trends) applied on oily or acne prone skin, can cause acne exacerbations.

Humectants attract water from the air or from deeper layers of the skin and help to retain that moisture in the skin. They come in three main forms: natural (not-altered), naturally derived, and synthetic. While humectants are most used in cosmetics and skin and hair care, they are often added to food products as anti-caking agents, and can also be found in some medications, and agricultural products.

EMULSIFIERS/SURFACTANTS

Since humectants are water soluble and emollients are lipid soluble, additional components are required to create homogeneity. These ingredients are emulsifiers.[21] Emulsifiers are surface-active agents which float within the interfaces between aqueous and oily phases and form links in between them. Simple cosmetic emulsions are classified as: oil in water (O/W), water in oil (W/O), water in silicone (W/Si), oil in water in oil (W/O/W), oil free, water free. These ingredients appear all along the INCI list, at different locations according to the concentration of its ingredients.

When used for skin cleansing purposes, these surface active agents are referred as surfactants.

PRESERVATIVES

Cosmetics, like any other product with expected shelf live, require preservation against contamination. The microbiological safety has two main goals: (1) consumer protection against potentially pathogenic microorganisms, and (2) product's preservation resulting from biological and physicochemical deterioration. These goals are achieved by combining synthetic or natural compounds in the formulation. The most popular ones include parabens and their derivatives, natural acids (search for the word BENZOIC and its derivatives in the INCI list, phenols and its derivatives), and so forth. Most preservatives are included in low percentages, so look for them at the end of the INCI list.[22] Recent study on cosmetic preservatives shows their unfavorable effect on the normal skin microflora.[23]

FRAGRANCES

Ingredients that are added to cosmetic products to provide a pleasant scent. Essential oils that are fragrance substances, are labeled in the INCI list by name of the specific extract. When the scent added to the formula, is extracted from a natural plant it may be called "natural fragrance additive," and thus patients who are allergic to it, will be not able to be specifically tested.[24]

It is important to note that not all cosmetic ingredients are safe for everyone.

SUMMARY

Skin care products are popular and currently used by virtually everybody. Skin specialists are required to consult their patients either regarding the benefits or to treat adverse effects, caused by these products. To address these needs, basic knowledge is required from the practicing dermatologists to read and understand the INCI list, labeled on the products as well as the basic principles of cosmetic products formulation.

CLINICS CARE POINTS

- INCI names of the ingredients are non -intuitive and can be be accessed via the Cosmetic Ingredient database (https://ec.europa.eu/growth/tools-databases-cosing.index.cfm?fuseaction=searc.simple)
- The ingredients of the cosmetic product appear in an order reflecting their concentration: the ingredients at the top oif the list are those with the highset concentration. Ingredients which concentration is lower than 1% do not appear in a particular order.
- While the foprmula of each cosmetic product may differ, most cosmetics contain a combination of at least some of the following core ingredients: excipients, additives and actives.

DISCLOSURE

The authors do not have any commercial or financial conflicts of interest and any funding sources for this work.

REFERENCES

1. Zirwas MJ. Contact Dermatitis to Cosmetics. Clin Rev Allergy Immunol 2019;56(1):119–28.
2. Groot AC, Weijland JW. Conversion of common names of cosmetic allergens to the INCI nomenclature. Contact Dermatitis 1997;37(4):145–50.
3. Draelos ZD, Gunt H, Zeichner J, et al. Clinical Evaluation of a Nature-Based Bakuchiol Anti-Aging Moisturizer for Sensitive Skin. J Drugs Dermatol 2020;1(12):1181–3.
4. Dhaliwal S, Rybak I, Ellis SR, et al. Prospective, randomized, double-blind assessment of topical

bakuchiol and retinol for facial photoageing. Br J Dermatol 2019;180(2):289–96.

5. Chaudhuri RK, Bojanowski K. Bakuchiol: a retinol-like functional compound revealed by gene expression profiling and clinically proven to have anti-aging effects. Int J Cosmet Sci 2014;36(3):221–30.

6. Lorencini M, Brohem CA, Dieamant GC, et al. Active ingredients against human epidermal aging. Ageing Res Rev 2014;15:100–15.

7. Saeedi M, Khezri K, Seyed Zakaryaei A, et al. A comprehensive review of the therapeutic potential of α-arbutin. Phytother Res 2021;35(8):4136–54.

8. Zaid AN, Al Ramahi R. Depigmentation and Anti-aging Treatment by Natural Molecules. Curr Pharm Des 2019;25(20):2292–312.

9. Boo YC. Mechanistic Basis and Clinical Evidence for the Applications of Nicotinamide (Niacinamide) to Control Skin Aging and Pigmentation. Antioxidants 2021;10(8):1315.

10. Ferreira MS, Sousa Lobo JM, Almeida IF. Sensitive skin: Active ingredients on the spotlight. Int J Cosmet Sci 2022;44(1):56–73.

11. Piątczak E, Dybowska M, Płuciennik E, et al. Identification and accumulation of phenolic compounds in the leaves and bark of Salix alba (L.) and their biological potential. Biomolecules 2020;29(10):1391.

12. Bassino E, Gasparri F, Munaron L. Pleiotropic Effects of White Willow Bark and 1,2-Decanediol on Human Adult Keratinocytes. Skin Pharmacol Physiol 2018;31(1):10–8.

13. Do NQ, Zheng S, Park B, et al. Camu-Camu Fruit Extract Inhibits Oxidative Stress and Inflammatory Responses by Regulating NFAT and Nrf2 Signaling Pathways in High Glucose-Induced Human Keratinocytes. Molecules 2021;26(11):3174.

14. Fracassetti D, Costa C, Moulay L, et al. Ellagic acid derivatives, ellagitannins, proanthocyanidins and other phenolics, vitamin C and antioxidant capacity of two powder products from camu-camu fruit (Myrciaria dubia). Food Chem 2013;139(1–4):578–88.

15. Enescu CD, Bedford LM, Potts G, et al. A review of topical vitamin C derivatives and their efficacy. J Cosmet Dermatol 2022;21(6):2349–59.

16. Madison KC. Barrier function of the skin: "la raison d'être" of the epidermis. J Invest Dermatol 2003 Aug;121(2):231–41.

17. Danby SG, Brown K, Higgs-Bayliss T, et al. The Effect of an Emollient Containing Urea, Ceramide NP, and Lactate on Skin Barrier Structure and Function in Older People with Dry Skin. Skin Pharmacol Physiol 2016;29(3):135–47.

18. Choi EH. Aging of the skin barrier. Clin Dermatol 2019;37(4):336–45.

19. Tagami H. Functional characteristics of the stratum corneum in photoaged skin in comparison with those found in intrinsic aging. Arch Dermatol Res 2008;300(Suppl 1):S1–6.

20. Verdier-Sévrain S, Bonté F. Skin hydration: a review on its molecular mechanisms. J Cosmet Dermatol 2007;6(2):75–82.

21. Scott GG, Börner T, Leser ME, et al. Directed Discovery of Tetrapeptide Emulsifiers. Front Chem 2022;17:10, 822868.

22. Halla N, Fernandes IP, Heleno SA, et al. Cosmetics Preservation: A Review on Present Strategies. Molecules 2018;23(7):1571.

23. Nasrollahi SA, Fattahi M, Khamesipoor A, et al. Effects of Cosmetic Preservatives on Healthy Facial Skin Microflora. J Clin Aesthet Dermatol 2022;15(8):34–7.

24. Sabroe RA, Holden CR, Gawkrodger DJ. Contact allergy to essential oils cannot always be predicted from allergy to fragrance markers in the baseline series. Contact Dermatitis 2016;74(4):236–41.

Update on Chemical Peels

Marina Landau, MD[a],*, Fotini Bageorgeou, MD[b]

KEYWORDS

- Peeling • Superficial • Medium • Deep • Segmental • TCA • Phenol

KEY POINTS

- Chemical peels are used for cosmetic skin enhancement hand for some medical indications.
- Chemical peels are classified as superficial, medium and deep and are used according to the depth of the pathological process to be treated.
- Chemical peels have a long-lasting history of use, but new observations and publications deepen and extend the knowledge and use of this importanr procedure.

DEFINITION

Chemical peeling is a procedure used for the cosmetic improvement of the skin or for the treatment of some medical skin disorders. Chemical exfoliating agent is applied to the skin to destruct portions of it through a controlled wounding with subsequent regeneration and rejuvenation of its components.

Understanding of the science behind chemical peeling is still evolving while studies investigating the histologic and long-term effects of peels provide data to support the clinical observations.

HISTORY

Chemical peels have been used by ancient Egyptians, Greeks, and Romans for skin enhancement. Dermatologists pioneered skin peeling for therapeutic purposes since 1800s. They treated pigmentations and scars by using chemicals in different combinations and concentrations.[1,2] Histological studies supporting clinical results have been published on chemical peels by both dermatologists and plastic surgeons. The introduction of light-based technologies at the end of 20th century, allegedly decreased the demand for chemical peels, and yet according to the statistics published annually at the official web sites of scientific societies, chemical peels are steel among the first 5 most popular non-surgical procedures (www.plasticsurgery.org).

In 2012 International Peeling Society (IPS) was established by a group of dermatologists with vast experience in the field of chemical peels. IPS ever since advanced guidelines of care, promotes quality training and education in peeling methodology and techniques, supports basic and clinical research, and targets the awareness and recognition of their value among professionals and patients (www.peelingsociety.com).

CLASSIFICATION OF CHEMICAL PEELS

Chemical peels are divided into three categories according to the depth of the wound created by the peeling solution: superficial, medium, and deep. Superficial peels penetrate the epidermis only; medium-depth peels damage the entire epidermis and papillary dermis, while deep peels create a wound to the level of mid-reticular dermis.[3,4]

The depth of the peel depends on multiple factors, such as the chemicals used, their concentration, mode of application, skin condition, and so forth. There is a direct correlation between the depth of the procedure, the level of discomfort and post-peel rehabilitation time, risk for potential complications and intensity of overall skin improvement.

Authors do not have any commercial or financial conflicts of interest and any funding sources for this work. Both authors are active members of International Peeling Society (IPS) (no profit organization).

[a] Department of Plastic and Reconstructive Surgery, Shamir Medical Center, Be'er Ya'aqov, 2 Hahunit street, Herzliya, Israel; [b] Chemical Peeling Department, Andreas Sygros Hospital of Dermatological and Venereal Diseases, University Clinic, National and Kapodistrian University, 5, Dragoumi street, Athens, Greece
* Corresponding author.
E-mail address: dr.marinaclinic@gmail.com

Dermatol Clin 42 (2024) 13–20
https://doi.org/10.1016/j.det.2023.06.005

derm.theclinics.com

WHEN ARE CHEMICAL PEELS INDICATED?

Normal human skin has an inherent mechanism of renewal. Newly formed epidermal cells mature and move up from the basal to the corneal layer along a period of 28 days. The complex enzymatic process causes their separation and shedding from the epidermis to be substituted by younger cells. This is a normal peeling process of young skin.[5] As we age, this process becomes less efficient. As a result, the corneal layer thickens and the skin losses its natural luminosity. In addition, abnormal pigment deposits in the skin layers; fibroblasts function slows down, negatively affecting renewal of the intercellular matrix. External factors, such as sun exposure and smoking further deteriorate skin appearance.[6]

Chemical peels replace pathological components of the skin with younger and healthier cellular and acellular components. Peels are indicated in both cosmetic and medical skin conditions. Cosmetic indications include dull skin's appearance, uneven tone, dyschromia, and skin wrinkling.[7] Medical conditions that benefit from chemical peels include solar keratosis, active acne, dyschromia, acanthosis nigricans, precancerous skin lesions, acne scars, and so forth.[8–17] Chemical peels can be performed locally, such as in cases of periorbital pigmentation, perioral wrinkles, lips aging or deep glabellar line.[9–12] Segmental peels combine a different depth of peeling for different areas of the face according to the specific needs of each area.[13] In sequential peels different peeling agents are applied one after another to increase efficacy without increasing the risks.[14,15] Body peels require extra-caution, since off-face skin often heals poorly.[16]

PROPRIETARY OR COMPOUNDED?

Chemical peels solutions can be compounded pharmaceutically or purchased as ready to use preparations.[8,17–19] It is generally truth regarding superficial products. Deeper peels usually need to be compounded, unless provided as a part of the educational event.

Experienced peelers prefer to prepare their own solution, sometimes combining different concentrations of the ingredients for different skin areas. For beginners, proprietary peels are usually a safer choice.

PATIENT'S CONSULTATION AND SELECTION

When evaluating a patient for the peeling procedure, extensive medical history should be taken. The patient must be questioned about general health status, including skin disorders, medications, allergies, smoking, previous cosmetic procedures, recurrent herpetic outbreaks, keloid formation and so forth. While there are almost no absolute contraindications for superficial peels, deeper procedures require mentally stable patients with realistic expectations, willing to have downtime-associated procedure, and being able to follow up precisely and obediently all the postprocedural instructions.

Pregnant and lactating patients are peeled only in exceptional circumstances.[18] Darker phenotypes can be peeled after discussing the benefits of the peeling procedure against the risks of the postinflammatory hyperpigmentation. Any preexisting cardiac condition need to be cleared out with treating cardiologist before deep peels containing phenol. Modification of chronic medications is sometimes required before phenol peel. The concept of oral isotretinoin being exclusion criteria for chemical peels, has been recently challenged. On the other hand, frontal fibrosing alopecia, a newly described type of facial lichen planus, should be considered as contraindication for deeper peels. Prepeel skin preparation is advised using retinoic acid and tyrosinase inhibitors.

SUPERFICIAL PEELS

Superficial peels are indicated for mild acne and postacne, superficial dyschromia, textural changes, and for skin refreshment. Serial procedures are needed to achieve these goals and combination and home care products (cosmeclinicals) is recommended. Due to their superficial action, these peels are appropriate for all skin phototypes.[3]

Treatment with a superficial peeling agent induces gentle visible skin exfoliation. This does not usually occur, when using peels based on alpha hydroxy acids. Visible peeling is not a mandatory reaction to achieve full beneficial effect of the peeling. Yet, some patients feel disappointed after a peeling procedure with no visible skin desquamation.

Common superficial peel agents include alpha hydroxy acids, such as glycolic, lactic, mandelic, and pyruvic acids; beta hydroxy acid (salicylic acid); Jessner solution; retinoic acid, and trichloroacetic acid (TCA) 10% to 15%.

The ideal candidate for superficial peel is a patient with mild skin damage and dyschromia or active acne and postacne sequela, who is seeking for minimal recovery time and is willing to go through a serial treatment to achieve the desirable results. Superficial peels do not affect wrinkles or deep pigmentations. They can be used on the body for extrafacial medical or aesthetic indications.

ALPHA-HYDROXY ACID PEELS

AHA acids are widely known as fruit acids and constitute a family of organic carboxylic acids. They can be of natural or synthetic origin. The mechanism of their action includes a decrease in corneocytes adhesion, induction of signal transduction to increase synthesis of the collagen and glycosaminoglycans in the dermis in addition to antioxidant properties.

Glycolic acid has the smallest molecular weight of all AHAs, penetrates the skin easily and therefore is the most common AHA used. Glycolic acid peels are commercially available as free acids, partially neutralized (higher pH), buffered, or esterified solutions. The application of the solution is performed after de-fatting of the skin using q-tips, gauze pads or brash. The skin is covered with a thin layer of the product, and neutralization or thorough washing is performed once the skin achieves uniform erythema. If focal frosting is observed in any area before full-face erythema appears, immediate neutralization/washing is performed at this site to avoid adverse effects. It is recommended to start with low concentration of the acid (20–30%) and to increase its concentration and exposure time during the subsequent sessions, according to the skin reaction.

Treatment schedule includes biweekly to monthly sessions combined with home skin care products for effective epidermal barrier rehabilitation (cosmeclinicals).

Mandelic acid is the mildest AHA and is used as a peeling agent for sensitive skins.

It can be applied as a solution or a foam and washed/neutralized according to the skin reaction.[8] Usually, during subsequent sessions, skin resistance develops, to allow prolonged exposure to the peeling agent and even progression to a more active one, such as glycolic acid.

In general, AHA are pregnancy category B and considered safe during pregnancy and lactation due to negligible dermal penetration.[19]

SALICYLIC ACID PEELS

Salicylic acid (SA) is a beta hydroxyl acid. Because of SA's lipophilic and comedolytic effects, it is particularly effective for comedonal acne. It is well-known in dermatology due to its keratolytic properties. Its exfoliative activity on the epidermis is almost devoid of associated inflammation; therefore, this agent can be safely used on the skin types that are prone to develop postinflammatory hyperpigmentation (PIH).[20] SA peels are preferred by some practitioners over other superficial peels in cases of acne and PIH.[21]

The formulations of SA used for the peeling are 20% or 30% in ethanol (SAHA), or polyethylene glycol (SA-PEG), or in ointment base in up to 50% concentration (Pasta Unna).[22] PEG vehicle was developed to slow the delivery of SA, while simultaneously increasing its follicular penetration. Compared to SAHA, which causes skin desquamation after 2 days, SA-PEG does not create visible peeling.[23,24]

The treatment regimen includes 6 peels 2-4 weeks apart. After cleansing and de-fatting of the skin the solution is applied using cotton tipped applicator or gauze sponge. The patient usually experiences very mild burning sensation and some report on upper respiratory tract irritation. White precipitate of the salicylic acid appears soon after the solution application (**Fig. 1**). This "psedofrosting" can be wiped away and should not be confused with a real frosting. SA peels do not require neutralization.

Salicylism or salicylic acid intoxication is a rare complication of salicylic acid when applied on over 50% of the body skin in high concentrations (50%), or under occlusion, as was used to treat ichthyosis, and is not related to a peeling of small areas, such as a facial skin.[25] SA is pregnancy category C but can be used safely on limited areas.[26]

RETINOIC ACID PEEL

Retinoic acid ia vitamin A synthetic analog, with intranuclear activity and nearly neutral pH. All-trans retinoic acid or tretinoin peels cause minimal discomfort during application. Tretinoin 5% to

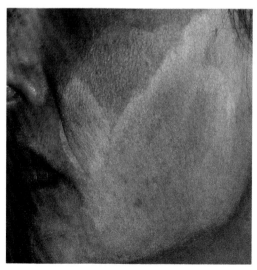

Fig. 1. A patient treated by salicylic acid 25% peel. Precipitation of salicylic acid on the skin is called pseudofrosting.

10% peels left on as a 6-hour facial mask cause mild erythema and desquamation on postpeel day 2.[27] Retinol peel 3% left for 8 hours was successfully used to treat aging signs and acne across a range of skin types.[28]

WHAT IS NEW?
Sequential superficial peels

Sequential peel is a procedure in which two different chemical agents/preparations are applied on the skin in the sequential mode. They intend to achieve better outcomes without increasing the associated risks, by using a more concentrated peeling agent. Sequential peels include, for example, a combination of 30% salicylic acid solution followed by the application of 3-5% retinoic acid cream. Despite scarce evidence to support their superiority, combination peels are currently a trend in chemical peels.

Warning regarding Jessner's solution

Jessner's solution has been used for the last century as a topical therapeutic agent for superficial peeling to remove hyperkeratotic layers of epidermis. Its use was first published in 1941.[29] Classical Jessner's solution is composed of 14% of salicylic acid, lactic acid, and resorcinol. Lately some concerns have been implicated to resorcinol medicinal use as a potential thyroid function disruptor as well as contact sensitizer.[30,31] Until more safety data is collected, Jessner's solution should be used with caution.

Combination of superficial peels with oral isotretinoin

Performing peels while on oral Isotretinoin used to be considered almost as a taboo. Recent publications demonstrate that the combination of oral Isotretinoin with SA based peels, improves patients' outcomes without increasing complication rate.[32,33]

MEDIUM-DEPTH PEELS

Clinical indications for medium-depth peels include dyschromia (mainly solar lentigines), multiple solar keratosis and textural changes of the skin (**Fig. 2**). Wrinkles and acne scars are improved only slightly, and usually deeper treatment modalities are required to provide more significant improvement in these cases.

TRICHLOROACETIC PEELS

TCA can be used in different concentrations. 35% TCA solution is used as a medium-depth peel agent. Concentrations higher than that, are not recommended, since the results are less predictable and the potential for scarring rises. To increase the efficacy of the TCA peel, without increasing the concentration of the acid, it has been suggested to precede this peel with Jessner's solution (Monheit's method), 70% glycolic acid (Coleman's method) or solid CO_2 (Brody's method).[21,22,34]

TCA solution is compounded as a weight to volume preparation. To prepare a 35% solution 35 g of TCA crystals are dissolved in water to make a

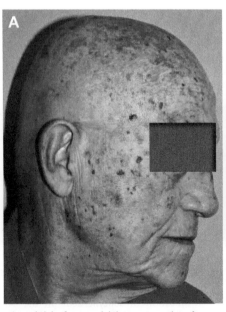
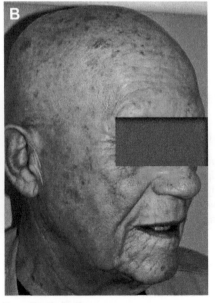

Fig. 2. A patient (A) before and (B) two months after medium-depth peel.

total volume of 100 mL.[24] TCA is stable in room temperature and is not light sensitive. It is nontoxic, non-allergenic, and self-neutralized.

TCA peel is a painful procedure. Therefore, oral or intravenous sedation, should be considered before the peel. The patient usually becomes completely comfortable 15-20 minutes after the procedure is finished, as the frosting subsides.

During the procedure of TCA is painted by q-tip or 4 × 4 gauzes, according to the cosmetic units until white frost appears. The degree of the frosting correlates with the depth of solution's penetration. While speckled white frosting with mild erythema corresponds to epidermal penetration, even white frost with background erythema points on superficial papillary dermis diffusion. Solid uniform white color usually characterizes the desirable depth of TCA procedure.

During the first days after the peel, patients are expected to feel tightening and swelling of the skin together with gradual crusting and darkening. On day 5 the skin starts cracking, and desquamation begins. Full re-epithelization is usually completed after 6-7 days. Medium-depth peel can be performed on the face and scalp skin exclusively.

TCA are pregnancy category N, and its use for cosmetic purposes during pregnancy should be discouraged. However, TCA has been safely used locally to treat genital condylomata in pregnant women.[35]

WHAT IS NEW?
Warning regarding Jessner's solution

Due to recent concerns, implicated resorcinol as a potential thyroid function disruptor and contact sensitizer, SAHA 30%, instead of Jessner's, can be considered for skin pretreatment when performing sequential TCA 35% peel.

DEEP PEELS

Main indications for deep chemical peel include dyschromia, fine and coarse wrinkles, premalignant skin tumors, and acne scars.[36] (Fig. 3) Deep peeling solution penetrates into the mid-reticular dermis and creates maximal effect on dermal fibroblasts to produce new collagen.[37,38] Occlusion increases the depth of effects when compared with unoccluded skin.[39,40]

The solution for deep peeling is composed of a combination of croton oil and phenol at different concentrations.[41] Phenol is an aromatic hydrocarbon derived originally from coal tar. Croton oil is an extract of the seed of the plant Croton tiglium, which causes skin vesiculation. Other chemicals in use in deep chemical peel formulas include septisol/novisol, water, vegetable oils (glycerin, olive, sesame), and so forth.

Cardiac safety is a concern for procedures involving more than 1 cosmetic unit, or more than 0.5% of the body surface area (equal to a palm without fingers). For peels exceeding 1% of the body surface area, intravenous hydration, continuous electrocardiographic monitoring, and ventilation/exhaustion of room air are recommended. The use of facial masks with activated carbon is recommended for the operating room personnel.

Intravenous sedation or regional blocks make the procedure pain-free. For the application of the peeling solution cotton-tipped applicators are employed. The usual end point is ivory-white to gray-white color of skin with foci of skin liquefaction.

Approximately 7% of patients undergoing full-face peels will exhibit transient intraoperative cardiac arrhythmias, which are more common in patients who are taking medications known to

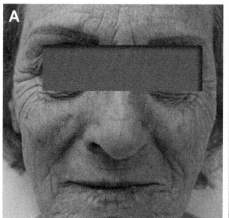
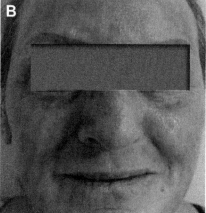

Fig. 3. A patient (*A*) before and (*B*) 3 months after deep peel.

prolong the rate-corrected QT interval, such as anti-hypertensive and antidepressant medications.[42,43]

If performing occlusive (deeper) peel, either waterproof zinc oxide non-permeable tape or occlusive moisturizers, antibiotic ointments, and biosynthetic occlusive dressings, can be used to deepen the solution penetration.

Full skin re-epithelization after deep peeling procedure usually occurs after 10-14 days, and the patient is advised to use water-based lotion creams and potent sunscreens. Postdeep peel erythema gradually subsides over a period of couple of months.

WHAT IS NEW?
Segmental peels

Segmental peels are used for non-synchronized facial skin aging. In such cases, different depths of a peel are targeted in different areas to address the specific pathology. For example, deep peel can be performed around the mouth or under the eyes, while the rest of the face is treated by medium-depth peeling solution.[44]

The advantage of this approach, when only a limited area is treated by phenol-croton oil solution, is easier and overall shorter rehabilitation with no need for cardiomonitoring during the procedure.[45]

Safety in darker phenotypes

PIH is one of the most important issues when performing deeper peels in darker phenotypes. Histologically, after phenol peel, melanin synthesis is impaired, accounting for the bleaching effect of a deep peeling procedure.[46] This effect is favorably accepted by dark skin patients.[45,46]

Deep peeling solution formulation

The original Baker- Gordon formula has been modified by Hetter, who proved in his work, that the major factor affecting peeling depth is croton oil concentration.[28]

By understanding this principle, phenol-croton oil solution composition can be modified to offer the ability to treat a variety of deep skin pathologies by strength gradation.

In 2020 the US FDA prohibited the use of triclosan. Triclosan was a component of Septisol, a necessary surfactant in Baker and Hetter's peeling solutions. Recently, Novisol has been suggested as an alternative to Septisol.[47] And yet, the recent publication suggests that the clinical endpoint when using Novisol might be different from when using Septisol.[48] It might be that the croton oil concentration in the formula containing Novisol, needs to be increased to achieve the same outcomes.[49]

New skin disorders, new possible contra-indications

Frontal fibrosing alopecia (FFA), that used to be a rare disorder of the hair in postmenopausal women, is currently considered as an emerging epidemic.[50] It proceeds with progressive fronto-temporal hair loss, but vellus hair follicles can be affected all over the face.[51] The etiology of the disease is unknown, and different genetic and environmental factors have been blamed, including sunscreens and some cosmetic procedures.[52] Intact follicles are required for normal skin healing after deeper chemical peels. Lack of bulge stem cells, negatively affects the postpeeling healing, increasing the risk of delayed erythema and scarring. At this point of time, we strongly suggest to consider FFA as contraindication for deeper peels.

SUMMARY

Chemical peels provide a diverse, powerful and yet non-expensive tool in medical and esthetic practice. The spectrum of conditions with a potential to benefit from peeling procedure is extremely broad. In spite of long-lasting history of use, new publications and clinical studies, deepen and upgrade our knowledge and understanding of this important procedure.

CLINICS CARE POINTS

- Chemical peels are usd for cosmetic enhancement of the skin but also for treatment of some medical skin disorders.

- Chemical peels are divided into superficial, medium and deep and are used according to the depth of the pathological process to be treated.

- Superficial peels are performed as serial in-office no downtime associated procedure.

- Some concerns have been recently implicated to resorcinol use as a potential thyroid disruptor and contact sensiizer.

- Trichloroacetic acid (TCA) 35% compounded as a weight to volume is a gold standard of medium depth peeling solution.

- Deep peeling solution is composed of a combination of croton oil and phenol. For peels exceeding 1% of the body surface area, intravenous hydration, continous electrocardiographic monitoring and ventilation/exhaustion of room air are recommended.

DISCLOSURE

None.

REFERENCES

1. Brody HJ, Monheit GD, Resnik SS, et al. A history of chemical peeling. Dermatol Surg 2000;26:405–9.
2. Borelli C, Ursin F, Steger F. The rise of chemical peeling in 19th-century European dermatology: emergence of agents, formulations, and treatments. J Eur Acad Dermatol Venereol 2020;34:1890–9.
3. Lee KC, Wambier CG, Soon SL, et al. Basic chemical peeling: superficial and medium-depth peels. J Am Acad Dermatol 2019;81(2):313–24.
4. Starkman SJ, Mangat DS. Chemical peel (deep, medium, light). Facial Plast Surg Clin North Am 2020; 28(1):45–57.
5. Has C. Peeling skin disorders: a paradigm for skin desquamation. J Invest Dermatol 2018;138(8): 1689–91.
6. Schumacher B, Krieg TM. The aging skin: from basic mechanisms to clinical applications. J Invest Dermatol 2021;141(4S):949–50.
7. Pathak A, Mohan R, Rohrich RJ. Chemical peels: role of chemical peels in facial rejuvenation today. Plast Reconstr Surg 2020;145(1):58e–66e.
8. Dayal S, Kalra KD, Sahu P. Comparative study of efficacy and safety of 45% mandelic acid versus 30% salicylic acid peels in mild-to-moderate acne vulgaris. J Cosmet Dermatol 2020;19(2):393–9.
9. Soon SL, Wambier CG, Rullan PR, et al. Phenol-croton oil chemical peeling induces durable improvement of constitutional periorbital dark circles. Dermatol Surg 2023;49(4):368–73. Epub ahead of print. PMID: 36735802.
10. Costa IMC, Peres AS, Costa MC, et al. Is there still a place for deep chemical peels in the treatment of perioral wrinkles? J Cosmet Dermatol 2020;19(10): 2634–6.
11. Wambier CG, Neitzke IC, Lee KC, et al. Augmentation and eversion of lips without injections: The lip peel. J Am Acad Dermatol 2019;80(5):e119–20.
12. Nogueira GC, Oliveira RIFM, de Queiroz MVR, et al. Static glabellar lines can be treated using a superlocalized phenol-croton peel. JAAD Int 2022;11:63–4.
13. Sterling JB, Lee KC, Wambier CG, et al. Depth Map for Face and Neck Deep Chemical Peel Resurfacing. Dermatol Surg 2020;46(9):1204–9.
14. Coleman WP 3rd, Futrell JM. The glycolic acid trichloroacetic acid peel. J Dermatol Surg Oncol 1994;20(1):76–80.
15. Monheit GD. The Jessner's + TCA peel: a medium-depth chemical peel. J Dermatol Surg Oncol 1989; 15:945–50.
16. Flynn TC, Coleman WP. Topical revitalization of body skin. J Eur Acad Dermatol Venereol 2000;14(4):280–4.
17. Lee KC, Wright M, Kulesza J, et al. Reviving the call for weight by volume standardization of trichloroacetic acid peel solutions. J Am Acad Dermatol 2020; 82(6):1542–4.
18. Garg AM, Mysore V. Dermatologic and Cosmetic Procedures in Pregnancy. J Cutan Aesthet Surg 2022;15(2):108–17.
19. Andersen FE. Final report on the safety assessment of glycolic acid, ammonium, calcium, potassium, and sodium glycolates, methyl, ethyl, propyl, and butyl glycolates, and lactic acid, ammonium, calcium, potassium, sodium, and TEA-lactates, methyl, ethyl, isopropyl, and butyl lactates, and lauryl, myristyl, and cetyl lactates. Int J Toxicol 1998;17:1–241.
20. Grimes PE. The safety and efficacy of salicylic acid chemical peels in darker racial-ethnic groups. Dermatol Surg 1999;25(1):18–22.
21. Lee HS, Kim IH. Salicylic acid peels for the treatment of acne vulgaris in Asian patients. Dermatol Surg 2003;29:1196–9.
22. Ueda S, Mitsugi K, Ichige K, et al. New formulation of chemical peeling agent: 30% salicylic acid in polyethylene glycol. Absorption and distribution of 14C-salicylic acid in polyethylene glycol applied topically to skin of hairless mice. J Dermatol Sci 2002 Apr;28(3):211–8.
23. Dainichi T, Ueda S, Imayama S, et al. Excellent clinical results with a new preparation for chemical peeling in acne: 30% salicylic acid in polyethylene glycol vehicle. Dermatol Surg 2008;34:891–9.
24. Dainichi T, Amano S, Matsunaga Y, et al. Chemical peeling by SA-PEG remodels photo-damaged skin: suppressing p53 expression and normalizing keratinocyte differentiation. J Invest Dermatol 2006;126: 416–21.
25. Brubacher JR, Hoffman RS. Salicylism from topical salicylates: review of the literature. J Toxicol Clin Toxicol 1996;34:431–6.
26. Bozzo P, Chua-Gocheco A, Einarson A. Safety of skin care products during pregnancy. Can Fam Physician 2011;57:665–7.
27. Magalhaees G, Borges M, Queiroz A, et al. Double-blind randomized study of 5% and 10% retinoic acid peels in the treatment of melasma: clinical evaluation and impact on the quality of life. Surg Cosmet Dermatol 2011;3:17–22.
28. Sadick N, Edison BL, John G, et al. An advanced, physician-strength retinol peel improves signs of aging and acne across a range of skin types including melasma and skin of color. J Drugs Dermatol 2019 Sep 1;18(9):918–23.
29. Fulton JE. Jessner's peel. In: Rubin MG, editor. Chemical peels. Philadelphia: Elsevier Saunders; 2006. p. 57–71.
30. Pasquier E, Viguié C, Fini JB, et al. Limits of the regulatory evaluation of resorcinol as a thyroid disruptor: When limited experimental data challenge

established effects in humans. Environ Res 2023; 222:115330.

31. IPCS, IOMC, WHO (2006) Concise International Chemical Assessment Document 71: Resorcinol. Available at: http://apps.who.int/iris/bitstream/handle/10665/43450/9241530715_eng.pdf;jsessionid=60EFD20D61D7682814BAC172D64B3D70?sequence=1. Accessed July 14, 2023.

32. Dixit N, Jena A, Panda M, et al. Randomized prospective study of low-dose isotretinoin alone and combination with salicylic acid and mandelic peel against acne tarda. J Cosmet Dermatol 2022; 21(10):4398–404.

33. Bs C, Vadlamudi SL, Shenoy C. Safety of performing superficial chemical peels in patients on oral isotretinoin for acne and acne-induced pigmentation. J Clin Aesthet Dermatol 2021;14(11):41–3.

34. Brody HJ, Hailey CW. Medium-depth chemical peeling of the skin: a variation of superficial chemosurgery. J Dermatol Surg Oncol 1986;12: 1268–75.

35. Lee KC, Korgavkar K, Dufresne RG Jr, et al. Safety of cosmetic dermatologic procedures during pregnancy. Dermatol Surg 2013;39(11):1573–86.

36. Wambier CG, Lee KC, Soon SL, et al. Advanced chemical peels: phenol-croton oil peel. J Am Acad Dermatol 2019;81(2):327–36.

37. Kligman AM, Baker TJ, Gordon HL. Long-term histologic follow-up of phenol face peels. Plast Reconstr Surg 1985;75:652–9.

38. Baker TJ, Gordon HL, Mosienko P, et al. Long-term histological study of skin after chemical face peeling. Plast Reconstr Surg 1974;53:522–5.

39. Spira M, Dahl C, Freeman R, et al. Chemosurgery- a histological study. Plast Reconstr Surg 1970;45: 247–53.

40. Stegman SJ. A study of dermabrasion and chemical peels in an animal model. J Dermatol Surg Oncol 1980;6:490–7.

41. Hetter G. An examination of the phenol-croton oil peel: Part I. Dissecting the formula. Plast Reconstr Surg 2000;105:239–48.

42. Landau M. Cardiac complications in deep chemical peels. Dermatol Surg 2007;33(2):190–3 [discussion: 193].

43. Wambier CG, Wambier SPF, Pilatti LEP, et al. Prolongation of rate-corrected QT interval during phenol-croton oil peels. J Am Acad Dermatol 2018;78(4): 810–2.

44. Lee KC, Sterling JB, Wambier CG, et al. Segmental phenol-Croton oil chemical peels for treatment of periorbital or perioral rhytides. J Am Acad Dermatol 2019;81(6):e165–6.

45. Sun HF, Lu HS, Sun LQ, et al. Chemical peeling with a modified phenol formula for the treatment of facial freckles on asian skin. Aesthetic Plast Surg 2018; 42(2):546–52.

46. Park JH, Choi YD, Kim SW, et al. Effectiveness of modified phenol peel (Exoderm) on facial wrinkles, acne scars and other skin problems of Asian patients. J Dermatol 2007;34(1):17–24.

47. da Silvo Justo A, Mikulis Lemes B, Nunes B, et al. Depth of injury of Hetter's phenolecroton oil chemical peel formula using 2 different emulsifying agents. J Am Acad Dermatol 2020;82:1544–6.

48. Kass LG, Rullan PP, Brody HJ. Clinical preliminary evaluation of PEG-80 sorbitan laurate (Novisol) versus triclosan (Septisol) in deep-peeling Hetter formulas. J Am Acad Dermatol 2020;82:e255–6.

49. Brody HJ. Commentary on 3 chemical peeling letters. J Am Acad Dermatol 2020;82(6):e257–8.

50. Mirmirani P, Tosti A, Goldberg L, et al. Frontal fibrosing alopecia: an emerging epidemic. Appendage Disord 2019;5:90–3.

51. Donati A, Molina L, Doche I, et al. Facial papules in frontal fibrosing alopecia: evidence of vellus follicle involvement. Arch Dermatol 2011;147:1424–7.

52. Di Petro A, Piraccini BM. Frontal alopecia after repeated botulinum toxin type A injections for forehead wrinkles: an underestimated entity? Skin Appendage Disord 2016;2:67–9.

Chemical Peels in Treatment of Melasma

Rashmi Sarkar, MD, FAMS[a],*, Saloni Katoch, MD[b,1]

KEYWORDS

- Chemical peels • Melasma • Glycolic acid • Salicylic acid • Trichloroacetic acid
- Jessner's solution • Tretinoin peel • Lactic acid

KEY POINTS

- Chemical peels are second-line therapeutic agents that primarily improve the epidermal component of melasma.
- Superficial peels like glycolic acid, salicylic acid, Jessner's solution, trichloroacetic acid, lactic acid, and tretinoin peel done serially have been found to be effective as additional or maintenance therapy.
- Medium to deep peels are not recommended in skin of color due to risk of post-inflammatory dyschromias and scarring.
- The choice of peel should depend on the skin type, expertise, and comfort of the treating dermatologist.
- Careful patient selection, counseling, pre peel preparation, and post peel care are essential components of patient management and play a vital role in the final outcome of melasma therapy.

INTRODUCTION

Chemexfoliation, chemabrasion, or chemical peels have been used since centuries for their rejuvenating and pigment diluting properties. The application of a chemical ablative agent to the skin surface causing controlled destruction of the epidermal or dermal layers followed by subsequent regeneration and remodeling has been in practice since ancient times.

The Egyptians used alabaster, salt, animal oils, and sour milk to improve the texture and appearance of their skin. Romans and Greeks used poultices made of sulfur, mustard, and limestone. A mixture of urine and pumice was used by Indian women. Similarly tree resins, fruits such as grapes, honey, and even fire have been used for aesthetic enhancement of the skin.[1] The history of modern chemical peel usage dates back to 1834 when skin peeling property of phenol was discovered by a chemist named Friedlieb Ferdinand Runge. In 1860, Ferdinand Hebra introduced the peeling properties of phenol in dermatology and treated melasma and freckles by using combinations of various exfoliative agents. Unna described the peeling properties of agents like salicylic acid (1882), resorcinol and trichloroacetic acid (1889).[2] Alpha hydroxy acids were used as superficial peeling agents in 1984 by Van Scott and Yu. This was followed by introduction of medium depth peels.[1] Currently as one of the most popular resurfacing procedures, chemical peels have shown efficacy in treatment of various hyperpigmentary disorders including melasma as an adjuvant therapy.

Melasma is a challenging hyperpigmentary disorder with symmetric light brown to brown hypermelanotic patches over the face with a chronic relapsing and recurrent course (**Fig. 1**). Treatment modalities are limited with topical applications like

[a] Department of Dermatology, Lady Hardinge Medical College and SSK and KSC Hospital, New Delhi 110001, India; [b] Dr. KN Barua Institute of Dermatological Sciences, Guwahati, Assam, India
[1] Present address: Dr. KN Barua Institute of Dermatological Sciences, 5th floor, Roodraksh Mall, Bhangagarh, Guwahati - 781005, Assam, India.
* Corresponding author.
E-mail address: rashmisarkar@gmail.com

Dermatol Clin 42 (2024) 21–32
https://doi.org/10.1016/j.det.2023.06.003

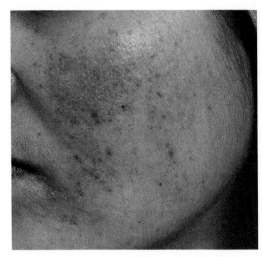

Fig. 1. Light to dark brown hyperpigmented patch of melasma over the malar region in an Indian patient. (Photo courtesy: Dr. KN Barua Institute of Dermatological Sciences, Assam, India.)

the triple combination cream and hydroquinone being the mainstay of treatment along with photoprotection. Other agents like glycolic acid, azelaic acid, kojic acid, arbutin, tretinoin, etc. have also shown efficacy in its management but the course of treatment can be prolonged often requiring long-term maintenance.[3,4] Management can often be frustrating for both the treating physician and the patient. With newer insights into the pathophysiology of this chronic condition and the realization that all melasma are of the mixed type with complex interplay between keratinocytes, melanocytes, dermal fibroblasts, and vascular endothelial cells, a multimodal treatment approach with various targets is found to be more beneficial.[5] Combination therapies with multiple topical agents (triple combination cream, dual combinations, etc.) or a combination of modalities (topical, oral, chemical peels, lasers) results in faster improvement, lesser side effects, and better patient compliance.[6,7] Chemical peels work effectively as second-line therapy, when combined with topical depigmenting agents resulting in rapid clearance of melasma and as an additional or maintenance therapy improve the overall efficacy of treatment.[7,8]

RATIONALE

A common acquired hypermelanotic condition, melasma usually affects women with Fitzpatrick skin type III-V with genetic predisposition, exposure to ultraviolet radiation, and hormonal influences affecting its variable course and chronicity. Research now suggests that along with epidermal

hyperpigmentation, dermal changes like solar elastosis and increased vascularity are also seen in melasma.[9] Dermal melanin may be present though its distribution has been reported to be very heterogeneous in the lesional skin.[10] Chemical peels form the second line of therapy in its management and help primarily in improvement of the epidermal component. By inducing controlled injury, the peeling agent causes epidermal dyscohesion and an accelerated keratinocyte turnover that has the following beneficial effects:[8,11–13]

- Melanin elimination from the epidermis and keratinocytes
- Epidermal remodeling
- Halting transfer of melanosomes to keratinocytes
- Inflammatory process leading to dermal reorganization
- Phagocytosis of stagnant melanin by macrophages improving the dermal component
- Cytokine production leading to an increased elastin and collagen synthesis

Chemical peels can be classified depending on their depth of penetration into the skin (**Table 1**).[14,15] Superficial chemical peels done serially can be used with mild to moderate efficacy as an adjunctive therapy in melasma.[7,8,11] Medium to deep peels should be used with extreme caution and are not recommended in dark skinned individuals due to the risk of post-inflammatory hyperpigmentation and scarring.[8,13,16] The outcome may vary depending on the type of peeling agent used, its concentration, number of coats, contact time, combination with other agents, pre peel priming, and post-procedure care.[8]

GENERAL PRINCIPLES
History

A thorough history and examination are a must in any patient of melasma undergoing a chemical peel. The duration of the condition should be noted as recent onset melasma responds better to peels. Any history of prolonged inadvertent usage of topical agents like triple combination creams and hydroquinone should be recorded as this may decrease peel tolerability and increase the risk of adverse effects. Drug history should also include oral isotretinoin intake in the past 6 to 12 months for medium and deep peels as this may interfere with wound healing. Photosensitizing drugs and oral contraceptive pills increase the risk of postprocedure hyperpigmentation. History of any skin infections like herpes simplex and dermatologic conditions like eczema, psoriasis, vitiligo, rosacea

Table 1
Classification of chemical peels based on depth of penetration[14,15]

Classification	Depth of Penetration	Examples	Suitability for Skin Type
Very superficial	Stratum corneum – 0.06 mm	30% glycolic acid (1–2 min) Jessner's solution (1–3 coats) 30% salicylic acid 10% trichloroacetic acid (1 coat) Lactic acid Phytic acid Tretinoin 1%–5%	Suitable in all Fitzpatrick skin types
Superficial	Up to epidermal basal layer – 0.45 mm	50%–70% glycolic acid 10%–25% trichloroacetic acid Jessner's solution (4–10 coats) 10% retinoic acid Mandelic acid Pyruvic acid	Suitable in all Fitzpatrick skin types
Medium	Up to papillary dermis – 0.6 mm	TCA 35%–50% TCA 35% + Solid Co2 TCA 35% +glycolic acid 70% TCA 35% + Jessner's solution	Ideal for patients with blue eyes and fair skin, Not suitable for skin types IV–VI due to risk of dyschromias and scarring
Deep	Up to midreticular dermis—0.8 mm	TCA 50% Phenol Baker–Gordon solution	Ideal for patients with blue eyes and fair skin, not suitable for skin types IV–VI due to risk of dyschromias and scarring

etc. that may worsen with the peel must be elicited. Any recent facial surgery should also be documented due to the risk of impaired wound healing. History of prior medium or deep peels in the past 3 months should be documented. Any coexisting systemic disease and comorbidity should be noted down as these patients can present with post-procedure infection and delayed wound healing. Adequate knowledge about the patients' hobbies and occupation with estimation of ultraviolet exposure plays a vital role in post peel recovery phase. History of pregnancy and lactation are vital in any woman of childbearing age.[8,14,15,17]

Examination

The patients' skin type must be assessed by using the Fitzpatrick phototype scale as skin color can aid in predicting pigmentary response to a peeling agent. This helps in patient selection as well as a guide for choosing a chemical peel. Evaluation of photoaging should be done with Glogau classification. The skin should be examined for erythema, dryness, erosions, signs of active infection, inflammation, and trauma. Co-existing dermatologic conditions that require treatment like acne, rosacea, topical steroid dependent skin, keloids, and hypertrophic scars must be assessed (**Fig. 2**). The severity of melasma can be recorded by using Melasma Area and Severity Index (MASI) score. This along with photodocumentation helps in pre- and post-treatment comparisons and evaluating response to therapy. Wood's lamp can be used to identify the predominant nature of hyperpigmentation (epidermal or dermal).[8,14,15,17] Dermoscopy when available can be a beneficial tool in diagnosis, classification, and assessment of treatment response in melasma patients (**Table 2**).[18–20]

Pre Peel Workup

The pre peel consultation should include an evaluation of the hyperpigmentation, counseling, and assessment of patients' motivation and

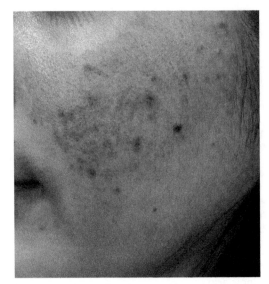

Fig. 2. A patient of melasma with co-existing acne and post-inflammatory hyperpigmentation. (Photo courtesy: Dr. KN Barua Institute of Dermatological Sciences, Assam, India.)

expectations from the procedure. A written informed consent must be taken after adequate discussion with the patient regarding the procedure, expected outcome, benefits, associated risks, and post-procedure care. Photographs must be taken at the first visit and can be repeated during subsequent follow-ups to document treatment

response. Patient selection is very crucial for a favorable outcome. Chemical peels are not indicated in melasma patients with unrealistic expectations, active infections, photosensitivity, prolonged duration, or a strong dermal component (visible clinically as gray brown or blue pigmentation). Superficial peels are safe to be used in all skin types but medium and deep peels should be avoided in skin of color as risk of scarring and dyschromias is high. Caution should also be exercised while treating male patients. With thicker, oily, and coarse skin, the peel penetration may be less predictable. A test spot may help in predicting pigmentary response, efficacy, complications, and healing time in medium and deep peels and can be done in less visible areas like the pre auricular region, lateral temple, and anterior hairline.[8,14,15,17]

Priming

The use of topical depigmenting agents for preparation of the skin before a chemical peel so as to ensure uniform and enhanced peel penetration and to decrease the risk of post-procedure complications is referred to as priming. This must begin at least 2 to 4 weeks prior to the chemical peel and should be stopped 2 to 5 days before the scheduled session. Pretreatment with priming agents also aid in detecting intolerability and in identifying noncompliant patients who are poor procedural candidates as they are less likely to follow post-

Table 2
Classification of melasma[18–20]

Melasma Type	Woods's Lamp	Dermoscopy	Clinical	Histopathology
Epidermal	Contrast enhancement seen	Regular network, homogeneous brown pigmentation, exaggerated pseudonetwork	Light brown-brown	Increased melanin in the basal layer and epidermis
Mixed	Contrast enhancement seen in some areas	Diffuse reticular pigmentation, Dark brown–gray brown, mixed features	Dark brown–gray brown	Increased melanin in epidermis and melanophages in dermis
Dermal	No contrast enhancement seen	Irregular pigment network with ash grey-bluish gray pigmentation	Bluish gray	Melanophages in the dermis
Wood's light inapparent (skin type V and VI)	Not evident	-	Ashen gray-unrecognized	Melanin deposition in dermis

procedure protocol. A broad-spectrum sunscreen with a sun protection factor (SPF) of 30 or above should be started at the patients first consultation. The patient should be advised to limit sun exposure and practice adequate photoprotection. This reduces melanocytic activity and reduces the risk of post-inflammatory hyperpigmentation. Ideally, sunscreens are to be initiated 3 months before the peeling session and should be continued long term thereafter. Topical agents used include 2% to 4% hydroquinone, 0.025% to 0.05% tretinoin, 5% to 10% glycolic acid, 1% to 4% kojic acid, and azelaic acid (**Table 3**).[8,15] Topical depigmenting agents can be restarted once the post peel desquamation is complete. Systemic antivirals must be prescribed for patients suffering from recurrent herpes simplex infection prior to medium or deep chemical peels.[8,14,15,17]

Post Peel Care

Post-procedure care is very essential for optimal skin recovery and prevention of complications. Patients must be counseled adequately about what to expect in the first few days after a chemical peel. Strict photoprotection with sunscreen application and sun avoidance must be advised after the peel. A bland emollient should be applied to prevent dryness and till the peeling is complete. Face must be washed with a mild nonsoap cleanser. Patients should also be instructed to avoid picking, scratching, or scrubbing their skin after the procedure. Makeup may be used once the skin reepithelization is complete. Patients should be educated about recognizing signs of complications (excessive redness, oozing, burning, pain, crusting, swelling, blister formation, purulent discharge) and reporting to the doctor so that timely action can be taken.[8,14,15,17]

CURRENT EVIDENCE

The most common chemical peels used for melasma include glycolic acid, salicylic acid, trichloroacetic acid (TCA), retinoic acid, and Jessner's peel.[8,11] There is also encouraging evidence for the use of newer peels like lactic acid, mandelic acid, lipohydroxy acid, amino acid, pyruvic acid, and phytic acid.[16,21]

Alpha Hydroxy Acids

These are fruit-derived acids that decrease keratinocyte adhesion at lower concentrations and are epidermolytic at higher concentrations. They require neutralization with water or sodium bicarbonate to terminate their action. The most common alpha hydroxy acid (AHA) used as an additional therapy in melasma is glycolic acid, which is derived from sugar canes. Lactic acid obtained from milk has also been reported to be effective. Other agents used include mandelic acid and phytic acid.[15]

Glycolic acid

A hydrophilic agent in the strengths of 30%, 50%, and 70% in gel base is used for melasma. The peel is applied for a duration of 3 to 5 minutes with 4 to 6 sessions done at 2 weekly intervals. Gel-based formulations are better suited for sensitive skin but higher amount of free acid is bioavailable in aqueous solutions with better cosmetic results.[8] Studies have reported an increase in overall efficacy in combination with topical agents like hydroquinone 2%, azelaic acid, and 0.025% tretinoin (**Fig. 3**).[7,22] Faster response has been reported with the addition of serial glycolic acid peels (30%–40%) to triple combination creams without any change in the overall efficacy.[23] Glycolic acid peel (70%) has been reported to have similar efficacy to 1% tretinoin peel, the latter being more tolerable.[24,25] In comparison to TCA peel, the efficacy was found to be similar with faster response and relapse in the TCA group.[26]

Lactic acid

Pure lactic acid (92%) was found to be safe and effective in a study, with 2 to 6 sessions at 3 weekly intervals.[27] The small molecular weight acid was reported to be as efficacious as Jessner's peel in another study.[28] Lactic acid (82%) applied only to the lesional skin, up to 2 coats and for a maximum of 10 minutes, 3 sessions at 2 weekly intervals was also reported to be effective in melasma.[29] In a comparative study 30% glycolic acid peel and 15% TCA peel were found to be more effective than 92% lactic acid peel. The lactic acid peel though was found to better tolerated by patients with minimum side effects.[30] Application of 82% lactic acid peel at 2 weekly intervals for a duration of 12 weeks has been reported to significantly decrease the MASI score in a study, with burning sensation as the only noted side effect.[31]

Mandelic acid

Due to its large size, mandelic acid penetrates the skin gradually and uniformly making this peeling agent well suited for sensitive skin.[14,16] Although its effects are subtle in comparison to glycolic acid peels, it has minimal side effects and lesser down time with complete reepithelization within 3 to 5 days allowing sessions at shortened intervals.[12] At concentrations of 10% to 50%, it can be used in melasma, at weekly or biweekly intervals. Its anti-inflammatory effects and synergism

Table 3
Common priming agents used for pre peel skin preparation[8,15]

Topical Agent	Priming Duration	Mechanism	Protocol Before and After Superficial Peels	Adverse Effects
Hydroquinone 2%–4%	4 wk	Reduces risk of post-inflammatory hyperpigmentation by reversible inhibition of tyrosinase enzyme and selective damage to melanocytes	Stopped 1–2 d before and restarted 1–2 d after the procedure	Irritant/allergic contact dermatitis, ochronosis
Tretinoin 0.025%–0.05% Can be used in combination with kojic acid, arbutin, or glycolic acid	2–4 wk	Thinning of the epidermis results in faster, uniform and deeper penetration of the peeling agent, also enhances epithelial differentiation and promotes re-epithelialization	Should be stopped 1–2 d before and restarted once peeling/desquamation is complete. Topical retinoids need to be combined with a good emollient as they can cause dryness	Dryness, irritation, increased photosensitivity, retinoid dermatitis
Glycolic acid 6%–12% Can be used in combination with tretinoin or hydroquinone	2–6 wk	Reduces epidermal cohesion facilitating penetration of active agents, increases keratinocyte turnover	Stopped 1 wk before and restarted 2–3 d after the procedure	Irritation, burning, erythema
Kojic acid More effective in combination with other agents	4 wk	Blocks tyrosinase activity by chelating copper	Stopped 1 d before and reintroduced 1 d after the peel	Sensitization potential

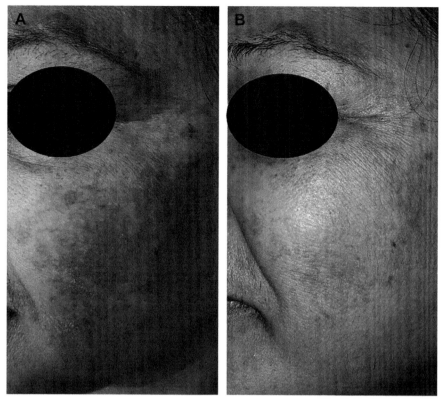

Fig. 3. Clinical images of a patient treated with oral antioxidants, strict sun protection, topical agents (retinoids and combination creams containing kojic acid, arbutin, licorice), and 4 sessions of a commercially available 44% glycolic acid combination peel. (*A*) Baseline photograph of the hyperpigmentation. (*B*) Improvement after 4 sessions of the peel done at monthly intervals. (Photo Courtesy: Dr. Meenaz Khoja, Consultant Dermatologist, Dermadent skin and dental clinic, Pune, India.)

with other peels make it an important agent in combination peels.[8] A combination peel with 20% salicylic acid and 10% mandelic acid was found to be as effective as glycolic acid 35%, safe and better suited for Indian skin.[32]

Phytic acid

A newer AHA with large molecular weight, antioxidant properties, and self-neutralizing action makes it more appropriate for sensitive skin. The peel can be done once weekly, with 5 to 6 sessions required to achieve lightening. Following application the peeling solution is left onto the skin until the next day.[14,16] This agent needs further evaluation with well-organized studies as it could be an effective peel in dark skinned patients. It is also commercially available as a combination peel with glycolic acid, mandelic acid, and lactic acid. The combination peel can be used at 2 weekly intervals, for 4 to 5 sessions in melasma.[8] Significant improvement in MASI scores was reported in Indian patients after 6 sessions with the phytic acid combination peel, at 2 weekly intervals in a

comparative study with glycolic acid (35%) and salicylic–mandelic combination peel, the latter 2 peels though were found to be more effective in melasma.[32]

Beta Hydroxy Acids

Salicylic acid

Salicylic acid is a beta hydroxy acid derived from natural sources like willow tree bark and wintergreen leaves. It is poorly soluble in water and has anti-inflammatory, keratolytic, antimicrobial, and analgesic properties. Widely used in acne, strengths of 20% to 30% have also been found to be useful as additional therapy in melasma. It dissolves intercellular lipids and is available in a polyethylene glycol or hydroethanol base.[15] In a comparative study on epidermal melasma in Asian skin, the efficacy of 30% salicylic acid peel and Jessner's solution was found to be similar.[33] Another study reported that 20% and 30% concentration of salicylic acid peel, 5 sessions at 2 weekly intervals is effective and safe in skin type V and VI for treatment of acne, melasma, postinflammatory hyperpigmentation, and oily skin.[34] The peel is applied for a duration of 3 to 5 minutes, leaves a white precipitate after evaporation of the base, and does not need neutralization.[15]

Lipohydroxy Acid

With an additional lipid chain and higher molecular weight, lipohydroxy acid (LHA) is a more lipophilic derivative of salicylic acid with a reservoir effect in the stratum corneum. Gradual penetration and the post peel exfoliation being similar to physiologic skin turnover make it more tolerable. Targeting the corneodesmosomal proteins makes it an excellent comedolytic and keratolytic agent. It also exhibits anti-inflammatory, sebostatic, and antimicrobial properties.[35,36] In a split face study with 5% to 10% LHA and glycolic acid (20%–50%) over a period of 9 weeks, significant improvement was reported in hyperpigmentation, fine lines, and wrinkles.[36] Nine patients (Fitzpatrick skin type II–IV) with superficial melasma underwent peeling with 10% LHA and 15% TCA with significant improvement in 67% of the patients.[37] Its application in melasma especially in ethnic skin needs more evaluation and research.

Trichloroacetic Acid

TCA is available in the form of hygroscopic crystals which when dissolved in water give a clear solution of the desired concentration. Its mechanism involves keratocoagulation which is clinically visible as frosting on the skin. The degree of frosting is used as a rough guide toward the cutaneous penetration of the acid (**Table 4**).[14] A strength of 10% to 30% works as a superficial peel, 35% to 50% as medium depth, and more than 50% as a deep peel. TCA can be used alone or in combination with other peels (**Fig. 4**).[14,15] The application of the peel requires expertise and caution even with lower strengths so as to avoid adverse effects like post-inflammatory hyperpigmentation especially in skin of color. The penetration of the acid increases with the number of coats. It does not need neutralization with frosting serving as the end point of the peel. TCA peel can be done once monthly, 4 to 6 sessions, with up to 2 coats on the lesional skin and 1 coat over the entire face.[8] TCA 10% to 20% was found to be similar in efficacy to different strengths of glycolic acid peel (20%–75%) in 2 studies, with faster response and relapses being more common with TCA. Glycolic acid was reported to have a better side effect profile.[26,38] Addition of topical agents like ascorbic acid to the peel regimen increases the overall efficacy and treatment outcome.[39] Modified Jessner's peel has also been found to be a useful adjuvant.[40]

Jessner's Solution

Jessner's solution formulated by Dr. Max Jessner is composed of 14 g of salicylic acid, 14 g of 85% lactic acid, and 14 g of resorcinol in ethanol. The modified solution instead of resorcinol contains 8% citric acid. Sessions are done at 2 weekly intervals, with 2 coats being applied for superficial peeling. Increasing the number of coats enhances the penetration and depth of the peel. Neutralization is not necessary with mild erythema being the end point.[8,14,15] A study found both Jessner's solution and 30% salicylic acid effective in melasma.[33] Modified Jessner's solution with 15% TCA was found to have improved results as compared to 15% TCA alone.[40] In a split face comparison, both 25% TCA peel and Jessner's solution were found to be effective in epidermal melasma with TCA being less tolerable.[41] Overall, Jessner's solution is an effective peel for hyperpigmentation when used alone or in combination with other peeling agents. It is

Table 4
Depth of cutaneous penetration and frosting patterns with trichloroacetic acid[15]

TCA Concentration	Level of Frosting	Depth of Cutaneous Penetration	Clinical Appearance	Use
10%–30%	I	Superficial	Mild erythema, speckled frosting pattern	Superficial peels
35%–50%	II	Medium	Background erythema with even white frosting	Medium depth peels, xanthelasma palpebrarum, chemical cauterization
>50%	III	Deep	No erythema, solid white frosting pattern	Xanthelasma palpebrarum, chemical reconstruction of skin scars technique, chemical cauterization

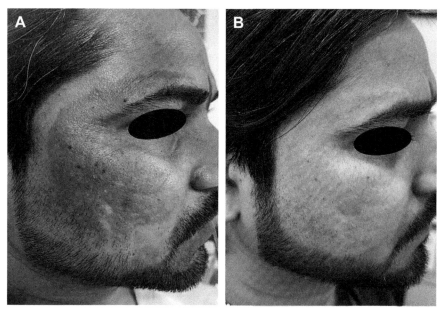

Fig. 4. Right lateral view of a patient of melasma treated with topical kojic acid, hydroquinone, oral tranexamic acid, and chemical peel sessions with a commercially available 15% TCA combination peel. (*A*) Clinical image of the patient before initiation of chemical peel sessions. (*B*) Significant improvement seen in the hyperpigmentation after 4 sessions at 3 weekly intervals. (Photo courtesy: Dr. Sonali Langar, Medical Director and Consultant Dermatologist, Skin remedies clinic and Laser centre, Noida, India.)

safe and effective in all skin types when used as a superficial peel.[8,16]

Tretinoin Peel (Retinoic Acid)

Tretinoin peel can be used in concentrations ranging from 5% to 12% as a stay on peel. It acts by melanin dispersion in the epidermis, stratum corneum thinning, and dermal remodeling. After application, the peel is left on for 4 to 24 hours followed by removal with water or a cleansing solution. It can be repeated weekly or monthly.[8,14] More organized studies are needed as the ideal concentration and vehicle for this volatile formulation still remain elusive.[11] In an Indian study, 1% tretinoin peel was found to be of equal efficacy to 70% glycolic acid peel. The peel was applied for 4 hours, once weekly for 12 weeks, the tretinoin peel was reported to be more tolerable.[25] In a study using a 10% tretinoin peel mask, significant improvement was reported in patients with melasma.[42]

Others

Amino fruit acid peels

These are acidified natural amino acids found to be beneficial in melasma due to their antioxidant, exfoliating, and pigment reducing properties. Because of its alkaline pH, amino acid peel is less irritating and is well suited for dry and

sensitive skin.[21] In a split face comparative study with glycolic acid peel, at 2 weekly intervals for up to 12 sessions, amino acid peel was found to be equally efficacious and better tolerated.[43] In combination with triple combination cream, amino acid peel was found to be effective in a patient of resistant melasma with satisfactory results.[21]

Pyruvic acid

Pyruvic acid is an alpha keto acid, which works via epidermolysis. It also has keratolytic, sebostatic, and antimicrobial properties. It also stimulates formation of collagen and elastin fibers in the dermis.[16] The peel is done with concentrations of 50%, 60%, and 80% in ethanol. After an application, the peel can be washed with water after 2 to 5 minutes of contact. Penetration of the acid sometimes can be quick and unpredictable; hence, this peel must be used with caution. Its vapors may also be caustic and irritant to the eyes and nose. Intense burning on application and post peel erythema, crusting, and desquamation have limited its use currently in many skin conditions.[14] Pyruvic acid in gel base is being reported to be better tolerated with the acid release being more gradual and uniform. Pyruvic acid 50% in a non-erythemogenic base, at 2 weekly intervals for up to 4 sessions was found to be safe and effective in treating melasma, photodamage, and superficial scarring in a study.[44] With most studies in patients with skin types II to IV, the safety and efficacy of pyruvic acid peel in melasma in ethnic skin needs more evaluation.

RECOMMENDATIONS

An evidence-based review with grades of recommendation concluded that all superficial peels can be used in melasma either as an additional or as maintenance therapy with mild to moderate efficacy. The use of glycolic acid peel was given a grade A recommendation, whereas other superficial peels like salicylic acid, lactic acid, TCA, tretinoin, and Jessner's peel were given a grade B recommendation. They also stated that chemical peels should be used by experienced dermatologists with selection of the peeling agent depending on the comfort and expertise of the treating doctor. They also concluded that no peel has been consistently found to be of superior efficacy than the other and that the safest strength of the peel should be used to avoid post-procedure complications.[7]

In contrast, due to the lack of good quality randomized controlled trials, chemical peels were not cited as a therapeutic modality in a recent network meta-analysis evaluating the efficacy of all available melasma treatment options.[45]

Various randomized and comparative studies on use of chemical peels in melasma were identified by Cassiano and colleagues[11] with several limiting factors like high heterogeneity, poor methodology, variable designs, small sample sizes, variation in selected population, types of peels, short-term follow-up, attrition rate, and deficient efficacy measures. They concluded that in melasma, glycolic acid peeling is safer and more effective than TCA peel. Jessner's peel and tretinoin peel were reported to be safe and cost-effective adjuvants. They also concluded that more well-designed studies are needed for evaluation of chemical peels in melasma.

SUMMARY

Melasma is a recurrent hyperpigmentary disorder with significant impact on the patients self-esteem and quality of life. As search continues for a safe, ideal, and curative modality of treatment, topical modalities like hydroquinone and the triple combination cream along with sun protection still continue to be the cornerstone of its management. Chemical peels are second-line therapeutic agents that primarily improve the epidermal component of melasma. Superficial peels like glycolic acid, salicylic acid, Jessner's solution, TCA peel, lactic acid, and tretinoin peel have been found to be effective as additional or maintenance therapy. The choice of

peeling agent should depend on the patients' skin type and comfort and expertise of the treating dermatologist. Various combinations of peeling agents are also commercially available in the market but evaluation of their safety and efficacy requires well-designed studies. A multimodal approach with topical agents, oral medicines, and chemical peels may result in faster response and improvement in the overall efficacy of therapy. Chemical peels are an important part of the dermatologists' therapeutic armamentarium against melasma with excellent cosmesis. Careful patient selection, counseling, pre peel preparation, and post peel care are also essential components and play a vital role in the final outcome of melasma therapy.

CLINICS CARE POINTS

- Patients must be advised to apply a broad-spectrum sunscreen adequately. Two finger strips of the sunscreen should be applied onto the face and repeated every 3 hourly between 9 AM and 4 PM.

- In the Indian scenario, melasma patients need to be assessed for side effects from inadvertent and prolonged usage of steroid and hydroquinone containing fairness creams. In such patients the steroid dependent skin will have to be treated first before considering any therapy for melasma. Once the skin sensitivity improves, well-tolerated peels like lactic acid can be considered.

- If a patient does not tolerate a priming agent (eg, glycolic acid), then it would be best to avoid using peels with such an agent (eg, glycolic acid peel) in these individuals to prevent adverse effects.

- Patients need to be counseled regarding the importance of post-procedure care with a bland moisturizer and physical sunscreen for optimal results.

- A minimum of 6 sessions with a superficial peel may be needed to see any visible improvement in the hyperpigmentation.

- If the melasma fails to improve after 6 sessions of any superficial peel, then one can consider that the pigmentation is primarily due to the dermal component. Other treatment modalities targeting the same should be considered.

- Medium and deep peels are not recommended in skin of color because of increased risk of post inflammatory hyperpigmentation.

- Monotherapy with chemical peels in melasma is not recommended.

- Adding a chemical peel to a patient's regimen also results in pan facial improvement and global rejuvenation, and this is probably the reason for the popularity of this procedure in a dermatologists' clinic.

DISCLOSURE

None.

REFERENCES

1. Brody HJ, Monheit GD, Resnik SS, et al. A History of Chemical Peeling. Dermatol Surg 2000;26(5):405–9.
2. Borelli C, Ursin F, Steger F. The rise of Chemical Peeling in 19th-century European Dermatology: emergence of agents, formulations and treatments. J Eur Acad Dermatol Venereol 2020;34(9):1890–9.
3. Bandyopadhyay D. Topical treatment of melasma. Indian J Dermatol 2009;54(4):303–9.
4. Sarkar R, Gokhale N, Godse K, et al. Medical Management of Melasma: A Review with Consensus Recommendations by Indian Pigmentary Expert Group. Indian J Dermatol 2017;62(6):558–77.
5. Sarkar R, Bansal A, Ailawadi P. Future therapies in melasma: What lies ahead? Indian J Dermatol Venereol Leprol 2020;86:8–17.
6. Ogbechie-Godec OA, Elbuluk N. Melasma: an Up-to-Date Comprehensive Review. Dermatol Ther 2017;7(3):305–18.
7. Sarma N, Chakraborty S, Poojary SA, et al. Evidence-based Review, Grade of Recommendation, and Suggested Treatment Recommendations for Melasma. Indian Dermatol Online J 2017;8(6):406–42.
8. Sarkar R, Arsiwala S, Dubey N, et al. Chemical peels in melasma: A review with consensus recommendations by Indian pigmentary expert group. Indian J Dermatol 2017;62:578–84.
9. Kwon SH, Hwang YJ, Lee SK, et al. Heterogeneous pathology of melasma and its clinical implications. Int J Mol Sci 2016;17:E824.
10. Kang HY, Ortonne JP. What should be considered in treatment of melasma. Ann Dermatol 2010;22:373–8.
11. Cassiano DP, Espósito ACC, da Silva CN, et al. Update on Melasma—Part II: Treatment. Dermatol Ther 2022;12:1989–2012.
12. Soleymani T, Lanoue J, Rahman Z. A Practical Approach to Chemical Peels: A Review of Fundamentals and Step-by-step Algorithmic Protocol for Treatment. J Clin Aesthet Dermatol 2018 Aug;11(8):21–8.
13. Chatterjee M, Vasudevan B. Recent advances in melasma. Pigment Int 2014;1:70–80.
14. Yokomizo VMF, Benemond TMH, Chisaki C, et al. Chemical peels: review and practical applications. Surg Cosmet Dermatol 2013;5(1):58–68.
15. O'Connor AA, Lowe PM, Shumack S, et al. Chemical peels: A review of current practice. Australas J Dermatol 2018;59:171–81.
16. Sarkar R, Bansal S, Garg VK. Chemical peels for melasma in dark-skinned patients. J Cutan Aesthet Surg 2012 Oct;5(4):247–53.
17. Anitha B. Prevention of complications in chemical peeling. J Cutan Aesthet Surg 2010 Sep;3(3):186–8.
18. Dharni R, Madke B, Singh AL. Correlation of clinico-dermatoscopic and Wood's lamp findings in patients having melasma. Pigment Int 2018;5:91–5.
19. Nanjundaswamy BL, Joseph JM, Raghavendra KR. A clinico dermoscopic study of melasma in a tertiary care center. Pigment Int 2017;4:98–103.
20. Sarkar R, Arora P, Garg VK, et al. Melasma update. Indian Dermatol Online J 2014 Oct;5(4):426–35.
21. Sarkar R, Chugh S, Garg VK. Newer and upcoming therapies for melasma. Indian J Dermatol Venereol Leprol 2012;78:417–28.
22. Garg VK, Sarkar R, Agarwal R. Comparative evaluation of beneficiary effects of priming agents (2% hydroquinone and 0.025% retinoic acid) in the treatment of melasma with glycolic acid peels. Dermatol Surg 2008 Aug;34:1032–9.
23. Sarkar R, Kaur C, Bhalla M, et al. The combination of glycolic acid peels with a topical regimen in the treatment of melasma in dark-skinned patients: A comparative study. Dermatol Surg 2002 Sep;28:828–32.
24. Faghihi G, Shahingohar A, Siadat AH. Comparison between 1% tretinoin peeling versus 70% glycolic acid peeling in the treatment of female patients with melasma. J Drugs Dermatol 2011;10:1439–42.
25. Khunger N, Sarkar R, Jain RK. Tretinoin peels versus glycolic acid peels in the treatment of melasma in dark-skinned patients. Dermatol Surg 2004;30:756–60.
26. Kalla G, Garg A, Kachhawa D. Chemical peeling—glycolic acid versus trichloroacetic acid in melasma. Indian J Dermatol Venereol Leprol 2001;67:82–4.
27. Sharquie KE, Al-Tikreety MM, Al-Mashhadani SA. Lactic acid as a new therapeutic peeling agent in melasma. Dermatol Surg 2005;31:149–54.
28. Sharquie KE, Al-Tikreety MM, Al-Mashhadani SA. Lactic acid chemical peels as a new therapeutic modality in melasma in comparison to Jessner's solution chemical peels. Dermatol Surg 2006;32:1429–36.
29. Sandin J, Oliveira TG, Curi VC, et al. Application of lactic acid peeling in patients with melasma: A comparative study. Surgical and Cosmetic Dermatology 2014;6:255–60.
30. Sahu P, Dayal S. Most worthwhile superficial chemical peel for melasma of skin of color: Authors' experience of glycolic, trichloroacetic acid, and lactic peel. Dermatol Ther 2021;34:e14693.

31. Singh R, Goyal S, Ahmed QR, et al. Effect of 82% Lactic Acid in Treatment of Melasma. Int Sch Res Notices 2014;2014:407142.

32. Sarkar R, Garg V, Bansal S, et al. Comparative Evaluation of Efficacy and Tolerability of Glycolic Acid, Salicylic Mandelic Acid, and Phytic Acid Combination Peels in Melasma. Dermatol Surg 2016;42(3):384–91.

33. Ejaz A, Raza N, Iftikhar N, et al. Comparison of 30% salicylic acid with Jessner's solution for superficial chemical peeling in epidermal melasma. J Coll Physicians Surg Pak 2008;18:205–8.

34. Grimes PE. The safety and efficacy of salicylic acid chemical peels in darker racial-ethnic groups. Dermatol Surg 1999;25(1):18–22.

35. Zeichner JA. The Use of Lipohydroxy Acid in Skin Care and Acne Treatment. J Clin Aesthet Dermatol 2016 Nov;9(11):40–3.

36. Rendon MI, Berson DS, Cohen JL, et al. Evidence and considerations in the application of chemical peels in skin disorders and aesthetic resurfacing. J Clin Aesthet Dermatol 2010 Jul;3(7):32–43.

37. Vavoulis C, Balamotis E, Kontochristopoulos G, et al. Efficacy and safety of lipohydroxy acid combined with trichloracetic acid facial peel. J Am Acad Dermatol 2013;P6943.

38. Puri N. Comparative study of 15% TCA peel versus 35% glycolic acid peel for the treatment of melasma. Indian Dermatol Online J 2012;3:109–13.

39. Soliman MM, Ramadan SA, Bassiouny DA, et al. Combined trichloroacetic acid peel and topical ascorbic acid versus trichloroacetic acid peel alone in the treatment of melasma: A comparative study. J Cosmet Dermatol 2007;6:89–94.

40. Safoury OS, Zaki NM, El Nabarawy EA, et al. A study comparing chemical peeling using modified Jessner's solution and 15% trichloroacetic acid versus 15% trichloroacetic acid in the treatment of melasma. Indian J Dermatol 2009;54:41–5.

41. Eyada MM, Abo bakr RA, El-Saman SF, et al. A Study Comparing Chemical Peeling using Trichloroacetic Acid and Jessner's Solution in the Treatment of Melasma. Suez canal University Medical Journal 2011;14(1):22–30.

42. Ghersetich I, Troiano M, Brazzini B, et al. Melasma: treatment with 10% tretinoin peeling mask. J Cosmet Dermatol 2010;9(2):117–21.

43. Ilknur T, Bicak MU, Demirtasoglu M, et al. Glycolic acid peels versus amino fruit acid peels in the treatment of melasma. Dermatol Surg 2010;36:490–5.

44. Berardesca E, Cameli N, Primavera G, et al. Clinical and instrumental evaluation of skin improvement after treatment with a new 50% pyruvic acid peel. Dermatol Surg 2006;32(4):526–31.

45. Liu Y, Wu S, Wu H, et al. Comparison of the efficacy of melasma treatments: a network meta-analysis of randomized controlled trials. Front Med 2021;8:713554.

Updates on Lasers in Dermatology

Ashaki D. Patel, MD[a,b],*, Rishi Chopra, MD[a,b], Mathew Avram, MD, JD[a,b],
Fernanda H. Sakamoto, MD, PhD[a,b], Suzanne Kilmer, MD[b,c], Richard Rox Anderson, MD[a,b],
Omar A. Ibrahimi, MD, PhD[b,d,1]

KEYWORDS

- Lasers • Dermatology • Updates • Vascular • Hair removal • Tattoo • Acne
- Selective photothermolysis

KEY POINTS

- Lasers can cause ablative or non-ablative tissue damage. When a laser is used to destroy only a single tissue target (or chromophore), it uses selective photothermolysis.
- Since the advent of selective photothermolysis, lasers have played a large role in expanding the capabilities of the procedural dermatologist.
- Selective photothermolysis allows for the precise and targeted treatment of many skin conditions.
- Fractional photothermolysis further expands the ability of procedural dermatologists to improve a variety of medical and cosmetic conditions.
- This review highlights how lasers have evolved since their introduction in the treatment of a variety of dermatologic applications.

INTRODUCTION AND HISTORY

The history of laser medicine starts with Albert Einstein's theory of stimulated emission, introduced in 1916. He postulated that when excited molecules/atoms interact with each other, they are able to stimulate emission of new photons that are of a similar frequency, phase, and direction as the original atoms/molecules. This concept was used by early physicists, including Theodore Maiman, to develop the earliest lasers. In 1963, Dr. Leon Goldman, a pioneer in laser medicine, first used a laser on human skin to treat melanoma. Dr. Goldman also used the continuous wave CO_2 and argon lasers to treat port wine stains.[1] Although the lesions he treated lightened, they had high rates of scarring and complications due to the non-selective nature in which the laser energy was absorbed in the skin. The theory of selective photothermolysis, as elucidated by Drs. John Parrish and Rox Anderson, propelled the use of lasers and forever changed the field of dermatology, and other medical specialties.[2] The concept of selective photothermolysis refers to localized, "selective," destruction of the desired target by combining a selective wavelength that is absorbed by the target chromophore and a pulse duration that is equal or shorter than the thermal relaxation time of the target chromophore. The combination of these 2 notions allows for more precise control of thermal energy and allows for more focused destruction. With the advent of selective

[a] Department of Dermatology, Massachusetts General Hospital Laser and Cosmetic Center, 50 Staniford Street, Suite 250, Boston, MA 02114, USA; [b] Wellman Center for Photomedicine, Massachusetts General Hospital, 15 Parkman Street, Wang Ambulatory Care Center - Suite 435, Boston, MA 02114, USA; [c] Laser & Skin Surgery Center of Northern California, 3837 J Street, Sacramento, CA 95816, USA; [d] Connecticut Skin Institute, Stamford, CT, USA

[1] Present address: 2 Hampton Road, Darien, CT 06820.

* Corresponding author. 3 Omni Drive, Schaumburg, IL 60193.

E-mail address: Apatel105@mgh.harvard.edu

Dermatol Clin 42 (2024) 33–44
https://doi.org/10.1016/j.det.2023.07.004

photothermolysis, the treatment of unwanted pigment, tattoos, and hair became possible. We went from non-selective lasers to early versions of both ablative and non-ablative lasers. Additional applications became possible with the advent of fractional photothermolysis.[3] The laser beam can be applied fully to the tissue, or it can be delivered in a pixilated pattern, called fractional photothermolysis (FP). FP can use both ablative and non-ablative wavelengths of light. This fractional injury is seen in the form of microscopic treatment zones (MTZ) that often form a grid pattern of injury on the skin. This allows for the sparing of normal tissue between each MTZ, and a shorter treatment recovery time. Interestingly, up to 50% of the tissue can be destroyed during FP without causing scarring or necrosis. By creating multiple laser holes in the skin, FP has been also used as a new method for drug delivery. This expansion continues with advances in technology and technique. Herein, we provide a review of updates in lasers as they are used in dermatology to treat a variety of medical and aesthetic conditions.

Vascular Lasers

One of the first applications of selective photothermolysis in dermatology was to help treat port wine stains.[4–6] Initially, the argon laser was introduced in the 1970s and was one of the first lasers used to treat port wine birthmarks (PWBs). These lasers functioned at a wavelength of 488 to 514 nm and although this wavelength is absorbed by hemoglobin in red blood cells, the thermal damage was not confined to the blood vessels but spread to adjacent tissue structures. Argon laser treatments caused significant scarring and were not an ideal treatment option for PWBs.[7] The pulsed deliver of the same wavelengths addressed these shortfalls and had fewer side effects, by allowing heat to diffuse strictly on the vessels. Earlier versions of the pulsed dye laser were 577 nm and worked well to selectively target blood vessels in port wine stains without significant thermal damage to the surrounding structures of the skin. However, as our understanding of laser-tissue interactions improved, so did technology. More recently, newer versions of the pulsed dye laser have larger spot sizes and a variety of pulse durations. This allows the dermatologic surgeon to treat lesions in purpuric and non-purpuric approaches. Having the option of larger spots sizes and more precise variation in pulse durations is advantageous because it allows for the treatment of certain vascular conditions, such as rosacea, with less purpura and downtime. The most recent previous version of the pulsed dye laser allowed for the

delivery of a maximum of 8 J with a maximum spot size of 12 mm. The newer pulsed dye laser has a larger spot size of 15 mm, allowing a maximum delivery of 12 J, an almost 50% increase as compared to the previous generation. This is important, as larger beam sizes allow for greater photon densities to be delivered at a greater depth, thus allowing more energy delivery to larger, deeper vessels in the skin. Additionally, the deeper penetration of energy allows bypass of epidermal melanin, reducing the risk of postinflammatory hyperpigmentation (PIH). The larger spot size also allows for broader surface area coverage and perhaps quicker treatment time. In 2021, Sodha and colleagues found that the larger spot size and safe delivery of increased energy allowed for shorter and fewer treatments to clear a port wine stain in 7 patients aged 10 to 38 years.[8] Even though the pulsed dye laser is considered the gold standard in PWB treatment, other various wavelengths of light have also been demonstrated to be useful in treating PWBs, especially those that are resistant to 577 to 595 nm wavelengths (**Fig. 1**). One reason lasers in the 577 to 595 nm wavelength may not be able to clear or even lighten a PWB is due to the depth of the penetration. PWBs are made of vessels of various depths. To reach deeper dermal vessels, longer wavelength lasers have been used such as the 755-nm alexandrite, 810-nm diode, and 1064-nm neodymium (Nd):yttrium-aluminum-garnet (YAG) lasers.[9] Additionally, in 2001, Barton and colleagues described how the combined effects of both green visible light and infrared wavelength light worked better to coagulate cutaneous blood vessels.[10] They described a synergistic phenomenon in which green light changes the constituents of blood to form methemoglobin, which then is better absorbed by infrared wavelengths. This led to the development of several laser systems that combined both wavelengths including a 595/1064 combination device, a 532/1064 device, and more recently, a 532/1064 device with variable sequential pulsing and cryogen spray cooling. Eichenfield and colleagues demonstrated the clinical effects of combining the 532 nm with 1064 nm wavelengths in treating vascular malformations in a cohort of 23 patients. They showed that combining these 2 wavelengths, 532-nm potassium titanyl phosphate to target superficial components and long-pulse 1064-nm Nd:YAG for deeper components, can safely and effectively treat both capillary venous and venous malformations.[11] However, the authors do not recommend treating capillary malformations and arterial vascular entities with 1064 nm, as the wavelength can often penetrate deeper and inadvertently select for deeper arterial

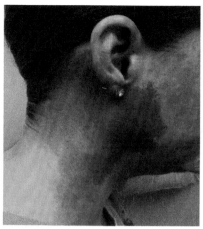 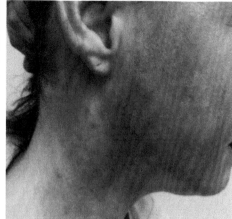

Fig. 1. Before and after 4 treatments of a port wine stain in an adult patient with a 595-nm pulsed dye laser. (*Courtesy of* Dr. Omar Ibrahimi.)

branches, leading to complications. Additionally, caution is also advised when treating venous entities with the 1064 nm wavelength as well, as the 1064 nm wavelength is more selective for oxyhemoglobin than it is for deoxyhemoglobin; therefore, sticking to the 755 nm wavelength is advised when treating older, more hypertrophic PWBs. Lastly, PWBs may be made of vessels of various diameters, requiring various pulse widths. A recent 532 nm/1064 nm combination device includes variable sequential pulsing with both sub-milli and sub-micro pulse modes, allowing for absorption by a broader size range of vessels.

In addition to revolutionizing how we treat vascular birthmarks, vascular lasers have also become standard of therapy for several other applications including angiomas, venous lakes, erythematous scars, and rosacea (**Fig. 2**).

CLINICS CARE POINTS

- Port wine stains typically take numerous treatments to lighten and complete removal is often challenging. Treatment should be initiated as early as possible as infants tend to respond better than adults.

- Treating within the bony orbit required the use of eye shields to protect the retina. While hemoglobin is the target chromophore, melanin is present in the retina and it also absorbs energy from most vascular lasers.

- Conditions such as rosacea can be treated with non-purpric settings and typically entail minimal downtime but require a series of treatments to bring about improvement.

Hair Removal

The most popular cutaneous application of laser energy is hair removal.[12] Laser hair removal (LHR) was first reported using a normal mode ruby laser and histologically showed selective destruction of the follicular shaft and epithelium.[13] The mechanism of action for LHR is unique in that the chromophore in LHR is the melanin found in the hair shaft, however, the intended target are the follicular stem cells found in the "bulge" and "bulb" of the hair shaft. Because of the small distance between where the melanocytes and stem cells are located, the extended theory of selective photothermolysis is used to fully describe the mechanism of action of laser hair removal. This theory suggests that there is some degree of diffusion of heat from the chromophore (melanin) and the desired target (stem cells).[14]

It is important to note that all devices for LHR target melanin as a chromophore and melanin is also present in the dermal–epidermal junction. Thus, some laser energy is absorbed into the epidermis and poses risk for adverse events such as burns, scarring, and postinflammatory dyspigmentation. A variety of methods for skin cooling have been developed to cool and protect the epidermal melanin and is a critical element in safely performing LHR procedures, especially when performed on darker Fitzpatrick phototypes. Cooling of the skin helps efface epidermal damage while also allowing treatment at higher fluences.[15] Most laser hair removal systems have built in cooling systems that act as heat sinks and help remove heat from the surface, either in the form of contact cooling with a cold sapphire or dynamic cooling with cryogen spray.

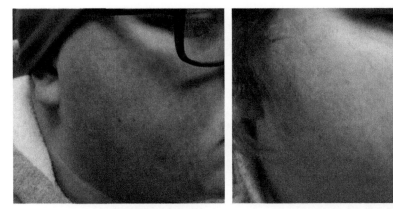

Fig. 2. Before and after 4 treatments for rosacea with a 595-nm pulsed dye laser. (*Courtesy of* Dr. Omar Ibrahimi.)

In addition to cooling, spot size is an important parameter in laser hair removal. Larger spot sizes allow more photons to be delivered to the target due to less scatter. Smaller spot sizes allow more scattering of photons. With less scatter and larger surface area covered, also minimizes the number of pulses required to cover a treatment area, thereby reducing treatment time. In one double-blinded, randomized controlled study, when all other treatment parameters are kept identical, an 18 mm spot size, as compared to a 12 mm spot size, led to 10% more reduction in hair counts.[16]

Today, there are multiple wavelengths available for LHR including 755 nm, 800 to 810 nm, and 1060 to 1064 nm (**Figs. 3** and **4**). Although long-pulsed ruby lasers are not commercially available in the United States, in one study, a majority of nearly 200 patients had >75% hair loss at the 6-month follow-up after 4 treatments.[17] Alexandrite and diode lasers, which are commercially available in the United States, showed similar results at about 76% to 84% at the 18-month mark for the Alex laser and 84% hair reduction at the 12-month mark for the Diode laser.[18,19] Although long-term hair reduction data are less convincing for the long-pulsed Nd:YAG laser at 1064 nm than other devices, this is thought to be the best wavelength for Fitzpatrick skin phototype V and VI.[20] A 1060-nm diode laser has also been recently reported to be safe and effective for LHR of all skin types, including darkly pigmented individuals.[21] The 1060 and 1064 nm wavelengths have much lower peak absorbance by melanin, making it less likely for epidermal melanin to be heated, and thus decreasing the risk of complications (see **Fig. 3**). Although intense pulsed light (IPL) is sometimes used for hair removal, IPL uses a flashlamp with broad band cutoff filter at different wavelengths that may not be as selective and deliver as much fluence as LHR. Therefore, one has to be careful, especially in treating darker skin types. Two studies that provide head-to-head comparison between the long-

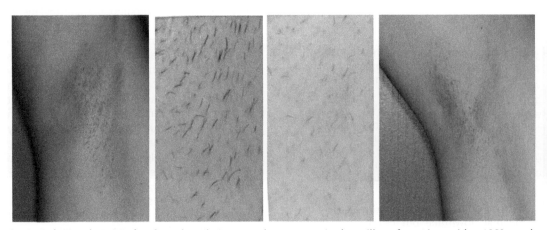

Fig. 3. Before and 15 months after 3 laser hair removal treatments in the axillae of a patient with a 1060-nm device. (*Courtesy of* Dr. Omar Ibrahimi.)

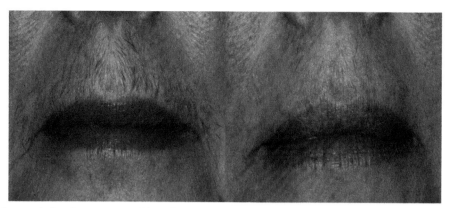

Fig. 4. Before and after 3 treatments of laser hair removal of the upper lip with a 755-nm device. (*Courtesy of* Dr. Omar Ibrahimi.)

pulsed Alexandrite and Nd-YAG found results from an IPL to be inferior.[22,23]

Prior to any treatments, it is important that clear expectations are set for the patient, and it should be communicated that LHR does not provide 100% *permanent* hair removal. Instead, there will be a significant permanent reduction in the growth of hair but there will be a few hairs which persist, though they are on average, 19% thinner and 10% lighter in color.[24] To help combat this problem, newer hair removal laser devices have the ability to deliver several long duration pulses in rapid succession such that the hair does not have the time to disperse the heat between pulses. The short delay between pulses is shorter than the thermal relaxation time of the melanin in the hair follicle being treated, and thus the hair does not cool off between the pulses, allowing for more damage to the hair follicle (patent). Although lasers in the 694 to 1064 nm range became the most effective way to achieve long-term hair removal, recently there have been devices that combine all 3 wavelengths for laser hair removal. In 2020 and 2021, 2 retrospective cohort studies showed that a simultaneous triple wavelength laser device is safe and effective.[25,26] The simultaneous triple-wavelength devices were shown to be safe in skin types III toV as well.[27,28] There are several devices that not only blend various wavelengths but also help deliver pulses at a programmed percent overlap. Lastly, along with advances in the technology itself, there have also been advances in procedure safety. In 2016, a group out of Massachusetts General Hospital used gas chromatography–mass spectrometry to analyze plume after laser hair removal and found several carcinogenic compounds within the plume and thus concluded that the plume should be considered a biohazard, warranting the use of smoke evacuators, ventilation, and respiratory protection.[29] In 2018, Ross and colleagues showed

that cold sapphire skin cooling suppressed plume from laser hair removal as compared to cryogen spray cooling, possibly eliminating the need for smoke evacuators, ventilation, and respiratory protection if using this method of cooling that required contact with a gel.[30] Nowadays, several newer lasers have built in smoke-evacuators to enhance user and patient safety.

CLINICS CARE POINTS

- Patients should be counseled that on average 15% of hairs will be removed with each laser treatment and treatments should be spaced about 6 to 8 weeks apart to allow hairs to properly cycle through the various growth phases.

- Avoid treating within the bony orbit, including the glabella, due to the high risk of retinal damage (the retina contains melanin dense tissues).

- Be careful to keep the handpiece perpendicular over convex and concave surfaces to ensure that the laser energy and any skin cooling methods are being delivered uniformly and will help avoid complications.

Tattoos

An important parameter within the theory of selective photothermolysis is laser pulse duration. Unlike the lasers used for vessels and hair removal, which are on the order of milliseconds, lasers designed for tattoo removal have optimal pulse duration in the order of picoseconds (**Figs. 5** and **6**). This is because the chromophore that is targeted in tattoo removal is tattoo ink, which is 10-

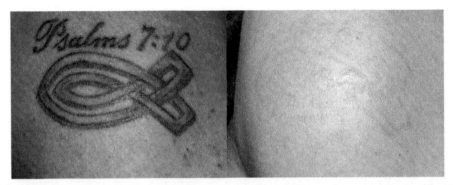

Fig. 5. Before and after 22 laser tattoo removal treatments with a 1064-nm picosecond device. (*Courtesy of* Dr. Omar Ibrahimi.)

4 to 10-3 mm wide. Based on this size, the pulse duration should be on the order of picoseconds. In 1998, Ross and colleagues tested this theory by comparing nanosecond domain pulses with picosecond domain pulses to remove black ink tattoos.[31] There was significantly more lightning with the picosecond laser pulses than the nanosecond laser pulses. In vitro studies show that picosecond lasers can remove smaller tattoo ink particles using lower fluences, and fewer number of treatments.[32] More recent human studies have corroborated this data and showed that, at matched fluences, picosecond lasers have been able to remove tattoos statistically more significantly than nanosecond lasers.[33,34] Today, picosecond lasers are considered the gold standard in tattoo removal. Conversely, long-pulse lasers and particularly IPLs, which also run in the millisecond domain, should not be used for tattoo removal, with a potential to cause severe scars.

In addition to pulse duration, successful tattoo removal depends on correct selection of wavelength. Colors in tattoo inks absorb the most visible light in the range of their complementary color. Based on this complementary matching of colors, green ink, for example, will be best removed by a laser that emits red light (694 nm). Some colors such as yellow and orange are more difficult to remove because there are few to no lasers on the market that operate in their complementary color ranges (400–520 nm).

However, tattoo removal remains a challenge even when using a picosecond laser in the correct wavelength range. There have been newer methods and technological developments that can be combined with picosecond.[35] A fractional ablative laser will allow extrusion of ink through the micro-columns that the laser creates.[35] Gas bubbles that are created during treatment with a picosecond laser can also escape faster through the micro-columns and thus allow for repeat passes. A recent study showed that the micro-focused arrays of a fractional nanosecond or picosecond laser allow for fewer treatments and more passes within 1 treatment session.[36] Alternatively, one can also do the fractional picosecond laser

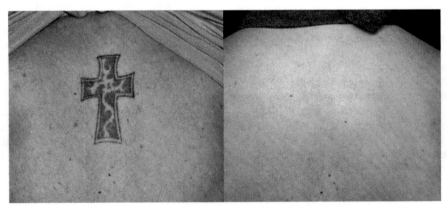

Fig. 6. Before and after 22 laser tattoo removal treatments with a 1064-nm picosecond device. (*Courtesy of* Dr. Omar Ibrahimi.)

after doing picosecond tattoo removal. Sirithana-badeekul and colleagues showed that this method allowed 84.6% of tattoos to be 50% cleared after multiple treatments versus 69.2% with picosecond laser alone.[36] Another shortcoming of tattoo removal has been that multiple treatments are required, even with picosecond lasers, to successfully lighten or clear a tattoo. In 2012, Kossida and colleagues reported that 4 passes of a Q-switched laser, separated by 20 minutes, was superior to a single pass treatment.[37] A waiting period of 20 minutes was necessary to allow the gas bubbles formed during picosecond laser treatment to fully dissipate before another pass of picosecond laser energy can be absorbed. This method of repeating treatments 20 minutes apart was dubbed the "R20 method." Given that the R20 method showed more clearance with a single pass, but took more time, the perfluorodecalin (PFD) patch was re-purposed for use in tattoo removal. PFD patches are silicon patches that contain fluorocarbon in them, a potent gas dissolver. Using this patch allowed for multiple laser passes in 1 treatment session without having to wait 20 minutes between sessions. PFD patches were shown to have other benefits as well, including limits in the increase of skin temperature during laser treatment.[38]

CLINICS CARE POINTS

- Laser tattoo removal requires matching an unwanted tattoo ink color to its complementary laser wavelength.

- Picosecond lasers are an improvement that has led to faster and better clearing of tattoos but most tattoos still fall short of complete clearance.

- Be cautious when treating a multicolored tattoo in the skin of color patient as melanin is targeted by many of the laser wavelengths used and can result in significant depigmentation and hypopigmentation.

- Newer, professional, and single ink color tattoos (ideally black) are easier to fade with laser treatments.

- The use of fractional ablative, repeat treatments, PFD patches, and rapid acoustic pulses may enhance and speed up laser tattoo removal.

- Never use a long pulse laser or an intense pulsed light (IPL) for tattoo removal, even if the device has the right wavelength for the color of the tattoo.

Pigmentation/Pigmented Lesions

Another way selective photothermolysis of melanin can be used in dermatology is for treating pigmented lesions. There are a wide variety of pigmented lesions in dermatology, and they vary in the amount of melanin deposition and/or increased density of active melanocytes. Common pigmented conditions that may be treated by lasers in dermatology include PIH, melasma, lentigines, café au lait macules, and nevus of Ota. There are occasional reports of lasers being used to treat more diffuse disorders of hyperpigmentation, including erythema dyschromium perstans, lichen planus pigmentosus, and drug-induced hyperpigmentation.[39–41]

Laser technologies have been extensively used to treat these benign epidermal and dermal pigmented lesions over the past 20 years since Anderson and colleagues first described the use of the Q-switched (QS) Nd: YAG laser to treat cutaneous pigmentation.[42] Although Q-switched lasers did provide some improvement in pigmented lesions, they produced high rates of PIH in certain skin types.[43,44] Picosecond pulses, however, are able to generate higher peak temperatures in a short amount of time, allowing for less unwanted heat diffusion. With picosecond pulses, lower fluences could be used for effective treatments, reducing the chances of PIH. Thus, more recently, picosecond lasers have played a huge role in our ability to treat individual pigmented lesions.[45] Many different wavelengths in the picosecond pulse duration range have been reported to safely treat pigmented lesions, ranging from 532 to 1064 nm.[46–49] Although picosecond lasers work well for individual lentigines, there have been several advances in near infrared wavelength resurfacing devices, which have allowed us to improve larger areas of pigmentation, including photodamage and even melasma. Since the introduction of the dual 1550/1927 nm fractional non-ablative laser, several variations in non-ablative technology have been released including the dual 1440/1927 low power diode laser, and the 1927 thulium laser. Each of these varies in power and downtime but can be paired with picosecond lasers for synergistic effects in treating pigmentation.

CLINICS CARE POINTS

- A proper evaluation of the pigmented lesion is needed prior to any laser treatments, ideally with dermoscopy.

- Lasers are not a first-line treatment for melasma. Melasma should be carefully evaluated and treated with first-line standard of care treatments to help stabilize pigment formation.

Scars

Lasers have also revolutionized how we treat scars in the past decade. In brief, injury to the skin triggers a multiphase healing process categorized into 3 main phases: inflammatory, proliferative, and remodeling. The proliferative phase occurs about 1 week post injury and is characterized by new vessel formation, fibroblast growth, and the creation of new extracellular matrix. During the remodeling phase, new collagen is being laid down, all while the scar is slowly decreasing its cellularity and vascularity to eventually build a mature scar.[50] In this long and tightly orchestrated chain of events, much can go wrong. Prolonged erythema, for example, can be an early sign of a pathologic scar. Vascular devices are often used to treat erythematous scars. Although we do not know the exact mechanism by which vascular devices are thought to help, there is some thought that the laser tissue interaction sets forth a cytokine cascade that triggers scar remodeling rather than simple vascular destruction.[51] Besides erythema, scar texture and thickness are also treatable via lasers. Fractional lasers, both ablative and non-ablative, are crucial in treating the spectrum of scars from atrophic to hypertrophic—the fractionated injury allows for remodeling of the scar without delivering too much thermal heat. Additionally, fractional lasers create microscopic treatment zones with cuffs of thermal coagulation. These channels are held open, due to the cuff of coagulation, and allow for subdermal delivery of topicals via a concept termed "laser-assisted drug-delivery"" (LADD). Ablative fractional lasers are a landmark treatment for hypertrophic scars in the last 10 to 15 years. In one consensus paper, 75% of the respondents use both a vascular and ablative fractional laser with or without LADD for thickened and/or contracted scars.[52] These lasers have been noted to allow improvement of texture, color, pliability, thickness, and quality of life.[53–56] Non-ablative fractional lasers have also shown to improve texture, specifically in hypertrophic and atrophic burn scars.[57,58] **(Fig. 7).**

CLINICS CARE POINTS

- Vascular lasers and fractional lasers (ablative and non-ablative) can treat a variety of scars with success.
- Be careful about laser parameters when treating scars. Treating at lower densities and higher pulse energies (depth) is safer for scars.
- It is never too late to initiate laser treatment for scars, though earlier treatment is better. Lasers can be implemented as early as right after wound formation. Complete epithelialization is not necessary to initiate laser treatment of scars.
- Although ablative fractional lasers can be used in darker skin types, one must tread with caution. In some circumstances, such as non-hypertrophic scars, non-ablative fractional lasers may be preferred over ablative to decrease the risk of PIH.

Acne

One of the newest applications of selective photothermolysis is for acne. Acne is one of the most

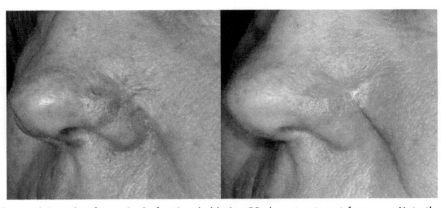

Fig. 7. Before and 6 weeks after a single fractional ablative CO_2 laser treatment for a scar. Note the improved texture, color, and thickness in certain areas. (*Courtesy of* Dr. Omar Ibrahimi.)

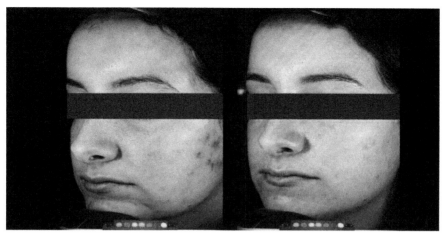

Fig. 8. Before and 24 months after a series of 4 monthly treatments with a 1726-nm device. (*Courtesy of* Dr. Emil Tanghetti & Accure Acne, Inc.)

common skin conditions worldwide, disproportionately affecting younger individuals. Although it is a very common condition, cure is difficult. Isotretinoin is an excellent oral option, but poses several side effects, compliance issues, and a minimum 6 months course on average. Additionally, many patients or parents are resistant to the use of isotretinoin. In the last decade, excellent developments have been made on targeting the sebaceous glands with selective photothermolysis as a hope to cure acne without the use of oral medications. In 2011, Sakamoto and colleagues described that both natural and artificial sebum had an absorption peak near 1,210, 1,726, 1,760, 2306, and 2,346 nm; however, laser-induced heating of sebum was approximately twice that of water at 1710 nm and 1720 nm.[59] Histologic skin samples exposed to ~1700 nm, with 100 to 125 milliseconds pulses, showed evidence of selective thermal damage to sebaceous glands.[59] At 1726 nm, the peak of absorption of acne sebum is about 30% higher than that of the surrounding tissue, making it possible to create a new acne-targeting laser by delivering high power (~40 W) with robust cooling (**Fig. 8**). Two new devices have been approved by the Food and Drug Administration (FDA) in 2022 to treat mild to severe acne and will likely forever change the way we approach the management of this common skin condition. In the FDA white papers, about 80% of inflammatory lesions were reduced in a multicenter study for both devices after 12 weeks of treatment, with sustained clearance for up to 2 years after 4 monthly treatment sessions. Even though both devices use the same wavelength, there are differences that might affect the overall efficacy and safety, but there are no comparative studies published to date.

CLINICS CARE POINTS

- Acne is the most common dermatologic complaint and complete cure remains elusive.
- Sebaceous glands are lipid rich and the development of a lipid-selective 1726 nm wavelength offers the ability to selectively damage sebaceous glands.

New Devices

Although there have been so many recent advances and updates in laser technology and its applications, there are continually new devices and applications in the pipeline. One promising development is a newer 3-dimensional (3D) laser that has been FDA cleared and will be commercially available in the United States soon. This 3D laser is highly focusable allowing laser energy to be targeted at precise depths in the dermis with reduced fluences at the epidermis. The reduced energy at the epidermis will make this a safer device for the skin of color patients. Additionally, there will be a high-resolution, high-speed imaging system that will be paired and integrated with the laser. This imaging system will not only allow mapping and guidance during treatment but also pretreatment and post-treatment skin changes to be archived, making way for a more personalized laser treatment for every patient.

Other devices modifications that may be on the horizon in the future include the integration of robots into dermatology. These laser "robots" may be programmed by humans, however, the action itself will be executed by robot software. Such a laser "robot" may be useful in skin cancer surgery, where we can perform image-guided laser ablation. Another way to integrate robots into lasers may be fractional-laser robots. These laser robots may be able to penetrate the skin at any precise depth and target several imageable structures such as sweat glands, nerves, cells, tumors, etc. These ablative fractional robot lasers may even be used for very precise drug delivery. The future remains very bright when it comes to the emergence of new technology that will advance our ability to treat a variety of medical and cosmetic dermatologic conditions.

DISCLOSURE

The authors have no disclosures to share (the authors need to look at disclosure criteria, certainly Rox, Fernanda, Mat, Suzy, and Ol may need to make disclosures). F.H. Sakamoto, science advisor for Accure Acne, Beiersdorf: receives portions of patent royalties from Massachusetts General Hospital.

REFERENCES

1. Goldman L, Dreffer R, Rockwell RJ Jr, et al. Treatment of portwine marks by an argon laser. J Dermatol Surg 1976;2(5):385–8.
2. Anderson RR, Parrish JA. Selective photothermolysis: precise microsurgery by selective absorption of pulsed radiation. Science 1983;220(4596):524–7.
3. Manstein D, Herron GS, Sink RK, et al. Fractional photothermolysis: a new concept for cutaneous remodeling using microscopic patterns of thermal injury. Lasers Surg Med 2004;34(5):426–38.
4. Kauvar AN, Geronemus RG. Treatment of port-wine stains. N Engl J Med 1998;339(9):635–6.
5. Goldman MP, Fitzpatrick RE, Ruiz-Esparza J. Treatment of portwine stains (capillary malformation) with the flashlamp-pumped pulsed dye laser. J Pediatr 1993;122:71–77 15.
6. Anderson RR, Parrish JA. Microvasculature can be selectively damaged using dye lasers: a basic theory and experimental evidence in human skin. Lasers Surg Med 1981;1:263–76.
7. Cosman B. Experience in the argon laser therapy of port wine stains. Plast Reconstr Surg 1980;65(2):119–29.
8. Sodha P, Richmond H, Friedman PM. Safe and Effective Use of a Novel Large Spot Size 595-nm Pulsed Dye Laser With High Energies for Rapid Improvement of Adult and Pediatric Port-Wine Birthmarks. Dermatol Surg 2021;47(8):1147–9. PMID: 33867471.
9. Izikson L, Anderson RR. Treatment endpoints for resistant port wine stains with a 755 nm laser. J Cosmet Laser Ther 2009 Mar;11(1):52–5.
10. Goldberg GN. Commentary on Efficacy and Safety of the 532-nm KTP and Long-Pulsed 1,064-nm Nd: YAG Laser for Treatment of Vascular Malformations. Dermatol Surg 2020;46(12):1540–1. PMID: 32604229.
11. Eichenfield, Dawn Z, Ortiz AE. Efficacy and Safety of the 532-nm KTP and Long-Pulsed 1064-nm Neodymium-doped Yttrium Aluminum Garnet Laser for Treatment of Vascular Malformations. Dermatol Surg 2020;46(12):1535–9.
12. Ibrahimi OA, Avram MM, Hanke CW, et al. Laser hair removal. Dermatol Ther 2011;24(1):94–107.
13. Grossman MC, Dierickx C, Farinelli W, et al. Damage to hair follicles by normal-mode ruby laser pulses. J Am Acad Dermatol 1996;35(6):889–94.
14. Altshuler GB, Anderson RR, Manstein D, et al. Extended theory of selective photothermolysis. Lasers Surg Med 2001;29(5):416–32.
15. Zenzie HH, Altshuler GB, Smirnov MZ, et al. Evaluation of cooling methods for laser dermatology. Lasers Surg Med 2000;26(2):130–44.
16. Nouri K, Chen H, Saghari S, et al. Comparing 18- vs. 12-mm spot size in hair removal using a gentlease 755-nm alexandrite laser. Dermatol Surg 2004;30(4 Pt 1):494–7.
17. Anderson RR, Burns AJ, Garden J, et al. Multicenter study of long-pulse ruby laser hair removal. Lasers Surg Med 1999;11(Suppl):11.
18. Davoudi SM, Behnia F, Gorouhi F, et al. Comparison of long-pulsed alexandrite and Nd : YAG lasers, individually and in combination, for leg hair reduction: an assessorblinded, randomized trial with 18 months of follow-up. Arch Dermatol 2008;144(10):1323–7.
19. Eremia S, Li C, Newman N. Laser hair removal with alexandrite versus diode laser using four treatment sessions: 1-year results. Dermatol Surg 2001;27(11):925–9. discussion 929–930.
20. Alster TS, Bryan H, Williams CM. Long-pulsed Nd: YAG laser-assisted hair removal in pigmented skin: a clinical and histological evaluation. Arch Dermatol 2001;137(7):885–9. PMID: 11453807.
21. Ross EV, Ibrahimi OA, Kilmer S. Long-term clinical evaluation of hair clearance in darkly pigmented individuals using a novel diode1060 nm wavelength with multiple treatment handpieces: A prospective analysis with modeling and histological findings. Lasers Surg Med 2018;50(9):893–901. Epub 2018 May 30. PMID: 29845623.
22. McGill DJ, Hutchison C, McKenzie E, et al. A randomised, split-face comparison of facial hair removal with the alexandrite laser and intense pulsed light system. Lasers Surg Med 2007;39(10):767–72.
23. Goh CL. Comparative study on a single treatment response to long pulse Nd : YAG lasers and intense pulse light therapy for hair removal on skin type IV to

VI – is longer wavelengths lasers preferred over shorter wavelengths lights for assisted hair removal. J Dermatolog Treat 2003;14(4):243–7.

24. Ibrahimi OA, Kilmer SL. Long-term clinical evaluation of a 800-nm long-pulsed diode laser with a large spot size and vacuum-assisted suction for hair removal. Dermatol Surg 2012;38(6):912–7. PMID: 22455549.

25. Lehavit A, Eran G, Moshe L, et al. A Combined Triple-Wavelength (755nm, 810nm, and 1064nm) Laser Device for Hair Removal: Efficacy and Safety Study. J Drugs Dermatol 2020;19(5):515–8. PMID: 32484620.

26. Noyman Y, Levi A, Reiter O, et al. Using blend wavelengths in order to improve the safety and efficacy of laser hair removal. J Cosmet Dermatol 2021;20(12):3913–6. Epub 2021 Oct 25. PMID: 34694683.

27. Gold MH, Biron J, Wilson A, et al. Safety and efficacy for hair removal in dark skin types III and IV with a high-powered, combined wavelength (810, 940 and 1060 nm) diode laser: A single-site pilot study. J Cosmet Dermatol 2022;21(5):1979–85. Epub 2022 Apr 6. PMID: 35306725.

28. Raj Kirit EP, Sivuni A, Ponugupati S, et al. Efficacy and safety of triple wavelength laser hair reduction in skin types IV to V. J Cosmet Dermatol 2021;20(4):1117–23. Epub 2021 Feb 22. PMID: 33567152.

29. Chuang GS, Farinelli W, Christiani DC, et al. Gaseous and Particulate Content of Laser Hair Removal Plume. JAMA Dermatol 2016;152(12):1320–6.

30. Ross EV, Chuang GS, Ortiz AE, et al. Airborne particulate concentration during laser hair removal: A comparison between cold sapphire with aqueous gel and cryogen skin cooling. Lasers Surg Med 2018;50(4):280–3. Epub 2017 Dec 7. PMID: 29214662.

31. Ross V, Naseef G, Lin G, et al. Comparison of responses of tattoos to picosecond and nanosecond Q-switched neodymium: YAG lasers. Arch Dermatol 1998;134(2):167–71.

32. Jang WH, Yoon Y, Kim W, et al. Erratum: Visualization of laser tattoo removal treatment effects in a mouse model by two-photon microscopy: publisher's note. Biomed Opt Express 2018;9(9):4162. Erratum for: Biomed Opt Express. 2017 Jul 20;8(8):3735-3748. PMID: 30615732; PMCID: PMC6157788.

33. Lorgeou A, Perrillat Y, Gral N, et al. Comparison of two picosecond lasers to a nanosecond laser for treating tattoos: a prospective randomized study on 49 patients. J Eur Acad Dermatol Venereol 2018;32(2):265–70. Epub 2017 Aug 21. PMID: 28758261.

34. Kono T, Chan HHL, Groff WF, et al. Prospective Comparison Study of 532/1064 nm Picosecond Laser vs 532/1064 nm Nanosecond Laser in the Treatment of Professional Tattoos in Asians. Laser Ther 2020;29(1):47–52. PMID: 32903983; PMCID: PMC7447827.

35. Ibrahimi OA, Syed Z, Sakamoto FH, et al. Treatment of tattoo allergy with ablative fractional resurfacing: a novel paradigm for tattoo removal. J Am Acad Dermatol 2011;64(6):1111–4. PMID: 21571169.

36. Sirithanabadeekul P, Vongchansathapat P, Sutthipisal N, et al. Outcomes of 1064-nm picosecond laser alone and in combination with fractional 1064-nm picosecond laser in tattoo removal. J Cosmet Dermatol 2022;21(7):2832–9. PMID: 35488471.

37. Kossida T, Rigopoulos D, Katsambas A, et al. Optimal tattoo removal in a single laser session based on the method of repeated exposures. J Am Acad Dermatol 2012;66(2):271–7. Epub 2011 Oct 27. PMID: 22036610.

38. Danysz W, Becker B, Begnier M, et al. The effect of the perfluorodecalin patch on particle emission and skin temperature during laser-induced tattoo removal. J Cosmet Laser Ther 2020;22(3):150–8. PMID: 32516063.

39. Wolfshohl JA, Geddes ER, Stout AB, et al. Improvement of erythema dyschromicum perstans using a combination of the 1,550-nm erbium-doped fractionated laser and topical tacrolimus ointment. Lasers Surg Med 2017;49(1):60–2. Epub 2016 Aug 23. PMID: 27552666.

40. Shah DSD, Aurangabadkar DS, Nikam DB. An open-label non-randomized prospective pilot study of the efficacy of Q-switched Nd-YAG laser in management of facial lichen planus pigmentosus. J Cosmet Laser Ther 2019;21(2):108–15. PMID: 29768073.

41. Barrett T, de Zwaan S. Picosecond alexandrite laser is superior to Q-switched Nd:YAG laser in treatment of minocycline-induced hyperpigmentation: A case study and review of the literature. J Cosmet Laser Ther 2018;20(7–8):387–90. Epub 2018 Feb 5. PMID: 29400580.

42. Anderson RR, Margolis RJ, Watenabe S. Selective photothermolysis of cutaneous pigmentation by Q-switched Nd:YAG laser pulses at1064, 532 and 355 nm. J Invest Dermatol 1989;93:28–32.

43. Wang CC, Sue YM, Yang CH, et al. A comparison of Q-switched alexandrite laser and intense pulsed light for the treatment of freckles and lentigines in Asian persons: A randomized, physician-blinded, split-face comparative trial. J Am Acad Dermatol 2006;54:804–10.

44. Chan HHH, Fung WKK, Ying SY, et al. An in vivo trial comparing the use of different types of 532nm Nd:YAG lasers in the treatment of facial lentigines in oriental patients. Derm Surg 2000;26:743–9.

45. Wu DC, Goldman MP, Wat H, et al. A systematic review of picosecond laser in dermatology: Evidence

and recommendations [published online ahead of print April 13, 2020]. Lasers Surg Med 2020. https://doi.org/10.1002/lsm.23244.

46. Guss L, Goldman MP, Wu DC. Picosecond 532 nm neodymium-doped yttrium aluminium garnet laser for the treatment of solar lentigines in darker skin types: Safety and efficacy. Dermatol Surg 2017; 43(3):456–9.

47. Chan JC, Shek SY, Kono T, et al. A retrospective analysis on the management of pigmented lesions using a picosecond 755-nm alexandrite laser in Asians. Lasers Surg Med 2016;48(1):23–9.

48. Alegre-Sanchez A, Jiménez-Gómez N, Moreno-Arrones ÓM, et al. Treatment of flat and elevated pigmented disorders with a 755-nm alexandrite picosecond laser: Clinical and histological evaluation. Lasers Med Sci 2018;33(8):1827–31.

49. Vachiramon V, Iamsumang W, Triyangkulsri K. Q-switched double frequency Nd:YAG 532-nm nanosecond laser vs. double frequency Nd:YAG 532-nm picosecond laser for the treatment of solar lentigines in Asians. Lasers Med Sci 2018;33(9): 1941–7.

50. Tredget E, Ding J. The cellular and molecular basis of scarring: the paradigm of hypertrophic scarring after thermal injury. In: Krakowski A, Shumaker P, editors. *The scar book*. Philadelphia: Wolters Kluwer; 2017. p. 104–8.

51. Kuo YR, Jeng SF, Wang FS, et al. Flashlamp pulsed dye laser (PDL) suppression of keloid proliferation through down- regulation of TGF-beta1 expression and extracellular matrix expression. Lasers Surg Med 2004;34(2):104–8.

52. Seago M, Shumaker PR, Spring LK, et al. Laser Treatment of Traumatic Scars and Contractures: 2020 International Consensus Recommendations. Lasers Surg Med 2020 Feb;52(2):96–116. Epub 2019 Dec 9. PMID: 31820478.

53. Blome-Eberwein S, Gogal C, Weiss MJ, et al. Prospective evaluation of fractional CO2 laser treatment of mature burn scars. J Burn Care Res 2016;37(6): 379–87.

54. Issler-Fisher AC, Fisher OM, Smialkowski AO, et al. Ablative fractional CO2 laser for burn scar reconstruction: An extensive subjective and objective short-term outcome analysis of a prospective treatment cohort. Burns 2017;43(3):573–82.

55. Anderson RR, Donelan MB, Hivnor C, et al. Laser treatment of traumatic scars with an emphasis on ablative fractional laser resurfacing: consensus report. JAMA Dermatol 2014;150(2):187–93.

56. Miletta N, Siwy K, Hivnor C, et al. Fractional ablative laser therapy is an effective treatment for hypertrophic burn scars: A prospective study of objective and subjective outcomes. Ann Surg 2019;274(6): e574–80.

57. Haedersdal M, Moreau KE, Beyer DM, et al. Fractional nonablative 1540 nm laser resurfacing for thermal burn scars: A randomized controlled trial. Lasers Surg Med 2009;41(3):189–95.

58. Waibel J, Wulkan AJ, Lupo M, et al. Treatment of burn scars with the 1,550 nm nonablative fractional Erbium Laser. Lasers Surg Med 2012;44(6):441–6.

59. Sakamoto FH, Doukas AG, Farinelli WA, et al. Selective photothermolysis to target sebaceous glands: theoretical estimation of parameters and preliminary results using a free electron laser. Lasers Surg Med 2012 Feb;44(2):175–83. Epub 2011 Dec 13. PMID: 22170298.

New Insight into Nonablative 675-nm Laser Technology
Current Applications and Future Perspectives

Martina Tolone, MD[1], Luigi Bennardo, MD[1], Elena Zappia, MD,
Elisabetta Scali, MD, PhD, Steven Paul Nisticò, MD, PhD*

KEYWORDS

• 675-nm laser • Melasma • Acne scars • Facial aging • Rejuvenation • Resurfacing

KEY POINTS

- The 675-nm laser has proven clinical effectiveness in the management of melasma, superficial melanosis, scars, and facial rejuvenation.
- The 675-nm laser, when used correctly, is associated with a very low incidence of side effects, mainly redness and superficial burning, that usually go away in couple of weeks.
- Given its histology and in vitro proven effect in stimulating collagen type III synthesis while not affecting cell viability and proliferation, this treatment may be used as a "rejuvenation" device, in order to reduce the loss of collagen during life.

INTRODUCTION

Laser devices are an exciting field of cosmetic dermatology.

Since the discovery of lasers in 1960s, more and more different lasers have been studied and launched on the market with a variety of applications. In medicine, different lasers have been proposed, mainly with a surgical and ablative purpose, in order to cut or vaporize tissues.[1,2] In dermatology and aesthetic medicine, however, a class of laser device, called nonablative lasers, with the purpose not to destroy tissues, but to convey energy in order to achieve a photobiological effect, has been proposed. These lasers, using a precise wavelength, have the goal to convey energy only to substances susceptible, using a theory called "selective photo-thermolysis." Thanks to this theory, every wavelength gets absorbed differently by the different substances contained in the skin (melanin, hemoglobin, water, and so forth), resulting in a different biological effect.[3–5]

For example, laser with a high-peak absorption for hemoglobin, such as 595-nm dye laser, is used in the management of vascular lesions, as well as lasers with high-peak absorption for melanin, such as 755-nm alexandrite laser, may be used for hair removal or in q-switched mode for the management of hyperpigmented lesions or tattoos.[6]

It is of course hard to discover a medium that generates a specific wavelength, so each time a specific laser with a specific wavelength is discovered, various studies are performed, in vitro and then in vivo, to find the possible clinical indications.[7,8]

Department of Health Sciences, Magna Graecia University, Catanzaro 88100, Italy
[1] These authors equally contributed to the article.
* Corresponding author. Department of Health Sciences, Magna Graecia University, Viale Europa SNC, Catanzaro 88100, Italy.
E-mail address: nistico@unicz.it

Dermatol Clin 42 (2024) 45–50
https://doi.org/10.1016/j.det.2023.06.004

Among the newly discovered lasers, the 675-nm diode laser (RedTouch, DEKA M.E.L.A., Calenzano, Italy) has become a more and more interesting device in cosmetic dermatology; at 675 nm, energy gets absorbed by dermal collagen and partially by melanin.

Thanks to a scanning system of 15 × 15 mm, the delivered energy can be managed through different parameters (power, pulse duration, and distance between microthermal zones).

The system is equipped with a contact 5 (degrees) C skin cooling system to preserve the epidermis from heat-induced damage.

In this article, the authors review all currently present medical literature regarding clinical use of this new emerging nonablative laser.

MATERIALS AND METHODS

The authors followed the criteria established in the preferred reporting items for systematic reviews and meta-analyses (PRISMA) guidelines for this review.[9]

A comprehensive literature search to identify relevant studies was carried out from the January 1, 2023 to April 15, 2023 using the following databases: MEDLINE/PubMed (National Center for Biotechnology Information, NCBI), EMBASE (Ovid), Google Scholar, and the Cochrane Central Register of Controlled Trials (CENTRAL). The keywords used to select the maximum number of pertinent studies included: "675 nm laser", "675 nm", and "675 nm emission". In addition, a search for citations in the reference lists of the selected articles and reviews was conducted to identify potentially missing studies.

Inclusion and Exclusion Criteria

The (PRISMA) methodology selected studies based on the following criteria. Only studies that met the following inclusion criteria were included: (a) Papers in the English language, and (b) all cited studies must have been approved by an ethics committee or an institutional review committee. Exclusion criteria were as follows: (a) papers that are not relevant, and (b) studies that do not provide sufficient data on the topic or when the paper was not available. The eligible articles were screened based on the title and abstract; finally, the full text of the articles that were potentially suitable for their inclusion in the review was analyzed.

In addition, the studies were rated using a modified Oxford Center for Evidence-Based Medicine 2011, and the levels of evidence were assigned to each association[10] (**Table 1**).

Table 1
Level of evidence for rating studies and grading recommendations (modified from[10])

Level	Type of Evidence
1°	Systematic review with homogeneity of randomized controlled trials
1b	Individual randomized control trial with a narrow confidence interval
1c	All-or-none related outcome
2°	Systematic review with homogeneity of cohort studies
2b	Individual cohort studies and low-quality randomized clinical trials
2c	Ecologic studies
3°	Systematic review of case-control or retrospective studies
3b	Individual case-control or retrospective studies
4	Case series and case reports
5	Expert opinion
Grades of Recommendation	
A	Consistent level 1 studies
B	Consistent level 2 or 3 studies or extrapolation from level 1 studies
C	Level 4 studies or extrapolation from level 2 or 3 studies
D	Level 5 evidence or contrasting results reported among studies

DISCUSSION

The 675-nm laser source is a new technology in the panorama of laser therapy with promising indications in the management of a large number of skin disorders.

Different clinical and preclinical studies indicate the ductility of this laser in managing connective tissue and melanin-based conditions.[11]

A preclinical histologic study showed that a 675-nm laser system produces selective skin thermal damage ("DOT" of 0.7-mm width) with an average depth of 500 μm, getting to the dermis. Compared with that in the untreated areas, the heating impact causes the denaturation of collagen fibers and the production of new collagen in the treated ones.[12]

The action of the new 675-nm device on collagen is also confirmed by in vitro studies. Magni and colleagues[13] analyzed adult Human Dermal Fibroblast cells post-675-nm laser irradiation doses. Fluorescence quantification showed a significant decrease in type I collagen combined with a significant increase in type III collagen. No dose tested showed effects on cell viability and proliferation.

The high affinity for collagen leads the 675-nm laser system in promising facial skin rejuvenation.[14,15]

Piccolo and colleagues[16] provided real-life data reporting a case series of patients treated by 675-nm laser. All patients achieved an improvement in skin texture after the treatment.

The stimulation of dermal fibroblasts and the production of new collagen make the 675-nm technology promising also in strategy for the remodeling of acne atrophic scars.[17]

Moreover, the 675-nm laser device shows a high affinity for the melanin chromophore. Both preclinical and clinical studies demonstrated its efficacy in the treatment of melasma, as reported by Nisticò and colleagues.[11]

These results have been confirmed also in Fitzpatrick phototypes IV to V.[18]

The strength of this treatment is that it is well-tolerated. Only minor erythematous-vesicular side effects, that resolve in a few days, have been reported in the literature. Posttreatment management is simple and includes moisturizer, physical sunblock, and hydrocortisone combined with fusidic acid in the case of minor burn.[11–14]

RESULTS

Only 8 studies met the inclusion criteria and were included in the review (**Table 2**).

What emerges in the literature is that this laser system was created primarily for the treatment of skin disorders related to aging.[13–16]

Skin aging is a complex process whereby different mechanisms have been observed: solar exposure, cigarette smoking, medications, alcohol use, gravity, body mass index, work and mental stress, diet, and endocrinology status. In this context, quantitative and qualitative alterations of collagen and elastin fibers seem to play a key role.[19]

Normal skin has been observed to undergo age-dependent changes in total collagen content. It is mainly type III collagen that decreases leading to a progressively increased type I/III collagen ratio.

These changes are superimposable if healthy and scarred skin are compared. Therefore, it can be said that, with advancing age, there is a progressive formation of scarlike tissue in the skin.[20]

Cannarozzo and colleagues[12] reported a 42-year-old man that underwent a 675-nm laser for the treatment of aging signs on his neck. Forty-five days after the procedure, a skin biopsy, taken from the treated area, and compared with ones of the adjacent area untreated with the laser, revealed histologic changes that comprised proliferation of thin and new collagen fibers in the treated area.

Moreover, in vitro studies have shown that the use of the 675-nm laser increases the amount of type III collagen in the areas undergoing treatment, restoring the collagen I/III collagen ratio in favor of the collagen type III.[13]

Therefore, the histologic findings and immuno-fluorescence analysis certify an important action of the 675-nm technology in the treatment of age-related skin disorders and allow its wide use in the field of skin rejuvenation.[12,13]

Clinical Studies

A prospective observational study conducted on 22 female subjects affected by facial wrinkles confirmed the clinical efficacy of the 675-nm laser in facial rejuvenation. A reduction of the wrinkles, objectified by the evaluation of the Modified Fitzpatrick Wrinkles Scale performed before and after 3 treatment sessions, was demonstrated in 100% of cases.[14]

Its efficacy in skin rejuvenation has also been successfully tested in the Asian phenotype.[15]

The results obtained by Piccolo and colleagues[16] confirmed the effectiveness of the 675-nm laser in reducing skin wrinkles and improving skin texture, related to the stimulation of dermal fibroblasts to produce new collagen. An improvement in the structure of the skin was observed in all of the 29 patients who underwent treatment with 675-nm technology. In particular, an improvement in skin tone in the lower third of the face, so a reduction of puppet lines (lip lines) and a redefinition of the jaw area, as well as a tensor effect of

Table 2
Skin disorders treated with 675-nm laser technology, associated level of evidence and grade of recommendation

Condition	References	Level of Evidence	Grade of Recommendation
Skin rejuvenation	2–6	III	B
Melasma	1,8	III	B
Acne scars	7	III	B

the zygomatic region with reduction of the nasolabial creases and an improvement in skin elasticity around the eyes, were observed.

Furthermore, the efficacy of the 675-nm laser in resurfacing is confirmed by the results obtained in the treatment of scarring in acne patients.[17]

Permanent scarring is one of the most distressing and long-term consequences of acne vulgaris that can have a negative impact on a patient's quality of life and is often worsened by aging.[21–23]

Different treatments are available to manage acne scars. Their treatment involves the use of different types of lasers: ablative (carbon dioxide laser, Erbium-YAG laser) and nonablative (Nd-YAG and diode lasers). Nonablative lasers stimulate dermal fibroblasts to produce new collagen, and in this context, the 675-nm technology is useful.[22,24]

An observational study enrolled 24 women (Fitzpatrick skin types I–IV) affected by residual acne scars evaluated by Goodman and Baron's Quantitative Global Acne Scarring Grading System (GBGS). All of the patients treated with 675-nm laser have an improvement of GBGS by comparing these score values before starting and at the end of treatment.[17]

The 675-nm wavelength acting both on collagen fibers and on melanin can also treat pigmented disorders and melasma.[25]

Melasma is a common hyperpigmentary disorder considered the consequence of hormonal stimulation and sun exposure on a predisposed genetic background.[26]

Its management is very difficult owing to 2 aspects, namely, the treatment resistance and the high recurrence rates.[27]

There are many possibilities to treat melasma, such as topical treatment: hydroquinone, tranexamic acid 5%, lignin peroxidase, petroselinum crispum solution, silymarin cream, and 4% diacetyl boldine serum, chemical peels (salicylic acid, glycolic acid, azelaic acid, ascorbic acid, phytic acid, mandelic acid, trichloroacetic acid, and Jessner solution), as well as systemic treatment: polypodium leucotomos, tranexamic acid, microneedling with a combination of tranexamic acid and glutathione, intense pulsed light; moreover, ablative lasers (fractional ablative CO_2 laser and nonablative lasers) can be successfully used.[28]

A prospective observational study was conducted on 25 women affected by facial melasma with both melanin and vascular component. Melasma severity was assessed clinically by comparing Multispectral Analysis Imaging System and measuring the Melasma Severity Index (MSI) score, before starting the treatment and at the 3-month follow-up after the last session. Twenty-two of 25 patients had a significant improvement in melasma. A mean 30% reduction of MSI (baseline [mean, MSI 26.4] to 3 months' follow-up after the last treatment [mean, MSI 17.3]) was observed.[11]

These brilliant results were confirmed by a study conducted on darker-skinned subjects with phototypes IV to V and affected by facial melasma treated with 3 sessions of the 675-nm laser. An objective evaluation was assessed by using a 5-point visual analog scale (VAS) for pain. A mean 3.1 ± 0.7 improvement was reached according to photographic evaluation by VAS. Patients treated 3 times showed a mean clearance of 3.0 ± 1.[18]

Although the 675-nm laser is effective overall in the treatment of facial rejuvenation, acne scars, and melasma, the treatments differ in terms of clinical outcomes depending on the patient's skin and the type of skin disorder.[11–14]

The superiority compared with the other available treatments for these 3 skin disorders has not yet been demonstrated, and further comparative clinical and/or histologic studies are needed for this purpose. The great advantage of this new 675-nm technology is its good tolerability. In all studies analyzed, the treatment was well tolerated by all treated patients. The pain assessed by the Pain VAS never seems to exceed 3/10 points. In terms of adverse events, only minor side effects have been reported consisting of small burns probably owing to incorrect positioning of the handpiece on the skin, with immediate resolution in less than 7 to 10 days.[11–14]

SUMMARY

Nowadays, laser technologies represent a valid therapeutic alternative for the treatment of many skin pathologic conditions. In the field of nonablative lasers, the 675-nm device demonstrated, initially in preclinical studies (histologic and in vitro) and subsequently in prospective observational clinical studies, its efficacy in the management of facial rejuvenation and in the treatment of acne vulgaris scars by promoting the synthesis of new collagen. Moreover, it is useful in the treatment of melasma by its ability to target melanin as well.

The outcomes are variable according to the patient and the pathologic condition treated. Further studies are necessary to establish its superiority in terms of efficacy concerning the other treatments and to ablative or nonablative laser technologies currently available for these 3 conditions. In terms of tolerability, however, the 675-nm laser appears to be safe and well tolerated. The reported side effects related to its use are only minor burns that can be managed with topical drugs and resolved in a few days.

A new concept of "pre-juvenation" is rising in cosmetic dermatology. This concept is based on the use of cosmetic procedures in order to preserve a youthful appearance starting from a very young age.[29] In this context, the use of a laser capable of increasing collagen production, with the lack of toxic effects, may be proposed in younger patients chronically or genetically exposed to photoaging.[13]

As regards to the prospects of this laser technology, it would be interesting to study its combined use with nonlaser treatments. In particular, evaluating their effectiveness in combination with injectables for face and neck rejuvenation could be stimulating and represent a great revolution in the field of aesthetic medicine.

CLINICS CARE POINTS

- The 675-nm laser has proven efficacy in the management of hyperpigmented benign lesions, scars, and photoaging (for all conditions, Level of Evidence: III, Grade of Recommendation: B).

- Given the low incidence of side effects (in all studies basically limited to redness and superficial burns), it may be useful to combine this device with other treatments, such as topical drugs and injectables, although no clinical studies are currently present in medical literature.

- 675-nm laser treatment may be useful also in young patients subject to photoaging, in order to block/delay the appearance of aging signs.

DISCLOSURE

The authors disclose no conflict of interest.

AUTHOR CONTRIBUTIONS

Conceptualization, M. Tolone, L. Bennaedo, and S.P. Nistico; validation, M. Tolone, L. Bennaedo, and S.P. Nistico; formal analysis, M. Tolone, L. Bennaedo; investigation, M. Tolone; data curation, M. Tolone, L. Bennaedo; writing—original draft preparation, M. Tolone, L. Bennaedo; writing—review and editing, L. Bennaedo, M. Tolone, and S.P. Nistico; visualization, M. Tolone; supervision, S.P. Nistico, L. Bennaedo. All authors have read and agreed to the published version of the manuscript.

FUNDING

This research received no external funding.

REFERENCES

1. Goldman L. Future of laser dermatology. Lasers Surg Med 1998;22(1):3–8.
2. Nistico SP, Silvestri M, Zingoni T, et al. Combination of Fractional CO2 Laser and Rhodamine-Intense Pulsed Light in Facial Rejuvenation: A Randomized Controlled Trial. Photobiomodul Photomed Laser Surg 2021;39(2):113–7.
3. Goldberg D, Kothare A, Doucette M, et al. Selective photothermolysis with a novel 1726 nm laser beam: A safe and effective solution for acne vulgaris. J Cosmet Dermatol 2023;22(2):486–96.
4. Ciocon DH, Doshi D, Goldberg DJ. Non-ablative lasers. Curr Probl Dermatol 2011;42:48–55.
5. Wang Y, Zheng Y, Cai S. Efficacy and safety of 1565-nm non-ablative fractional laser versus long-pulsed 1064-nm Nd:YAG laser in treating enlarged facial pores. Lasers Med Sci 2022;37(8):3279–84.
6. Cannarozzo G, Negosanti F, Sannino M, et al. Q-switched Nd:YAG laser for cosmetic tattoo removal. Dermatol Ther 2019;32(5):e13042.
7. Ganti SS, Banga AK. Non-Ablative Fractional Laser to Facilitate Transdermal Delivery. J Pharm Sci 2016;105(11):3324–32.
8. Lukac M, Zorman A, Lukac N, et al. Characteristics of non-ablative resurfacing of soft tissues by repetitive Er:YAG laser pulse irradiation. Lasers Surg Med 2021;53(9):1266–78.
9. Liberati A, Altman DG, Tetzlaff J, et al. The PRISMA statement for reporting systematic reviews and meta-analyses of studies that evaluate health care interventions: Explanation and elaboration. J Clin Epidemiol 2009;62:e1–34.
10. OCEBM Levels of Evidence—Centre for Evidence-Based Medicine, University of Oxford. Available online: https://www.cebm.ox.ac.uk/resources/levels-of-evidence/ocebm-levels-of-evidence. Accessed 13 February, 2021
11. Nisticò SP, Tolone M, Zingoni T, et al. A New 675 nm Laser Device in the Treatment of Melasma: Results of a Prospective Observational Study. Photobiomodul Photomed Laser Surg 2020;38(9):560–4.
12. Cannarozzo G, Bennardo L, Zingoni T, et al. Histological Skin Changes After Treatment with 675 nm Laser. Photobiomodul Photomed Laser Surg 2021;39(9):617–21.
13. Magni G, Pieri L, Fusco I, et al. Laser emission at 675 nm: In vitro study evidence of a promising role in skin rejuvenation. Regen Ther 2023;22:176–80.
14. Cannarozzo G, Fazia G, Bennardo L, et al. A New 675 nm Laser Device in the Treatment of Facial

Aging: A Prospective Observational Study. Photo-biomodul Photomed Laser Surg 2021;39(2):118–22.

15. Bonan P, Verdelli A, Pieri L, et al. Facial rejuvenation: A safe and effective treatment with a fractional non-ablative 675 nm laser in Asian population. J Cosmet Dermatol 2021;20(12):4070–2.

16. Piccolo D, Kostaki D, Crisman G, et al. Resurfacing with a new 675-nm laser device: A case series. J Cosmet Dermatol 2021;20(4):1343–5.

17. Cannarozzo G, Silvestri M, Tamburi F, et al. A new 675-nm laser device in the treatment of acne scars: an observational study. Lasers Med Sci 2021;36(1):227–31.

18. Bonan P, Verdelli A, Pieri L, et al. Could 675-nm laser treatment be effective for facial melasma even in darker phototype? Photobiomodul Photomed Laser Surg 2021;39(10):634–6.

19. Prasanth MI, Sivamaruthi BS, Chaiyasut C, et al. A Review of the Role of Green Tea (*Camellia sinensis*) in Antiphotoaging, Stress Resistance, Neuroprotection, and Autophagy. Nutrients 2019;11(2):474.

20. Cheng W, Yan-hua R, Fang-gang N, et al. The content and ratio of type I and III collagen in skin differ with age and injury. Afr J Biotechnol 2013;10:2524–9.

21. Clark AK, Saric S, Sivamani RK. Acne scars: how do we grade them? Am J Clin Dermatol 2018;19(2):139–44.

22. Sadick NS, Cardona A. Laser treatment for facial acne scars: a review. J Cosmet Laser Ther 2018;20(7–8):424–35.

23. Chilicka K, Rusztowicz M, Szyguła R, et al. Methods for the improvement of acne scars used in dermatology and cosmetology: a review. J Clin Med 2022;11(10):2744.

24. Salameh F, Shumaker PR, Goodman GJ, et al. Energy-based devices for the treatment of Acne Scars: 2022 International consensus recommendations. Lasers Surg Med 2022;54(1):10–26.

25. Scholkmann F, Kleiser S, Metz AJ, et al. A review on continuous wave functional near-infrared spectroscopy and imaging instrumentation and methodology. Neuroimage 2014;85(Pt 1):6–27.

26. Passeron T, Picardo M. Melasma, a photoaging disorder. Pigment Cell Melanoma Res 2018;31(4):461–5.

27. Artzi O, Horovitz T, Bar-Ilan E, et al. The pathogenesis of melasma and implications for treatment. J Cosmet Dermatol 2021;20(11):3432–45.

28. Neagu N, Conforti C, Agozzino M, et al. Melasma treatment: a systematic review. J Dermatolog Treat 2022;33(4):1816–37.

29. Hogan SR, Zachary CB, Arndt KA. Prejuvenation: definition of the term and evolution of the concept. Dermatologic Surg 2021;47:871–2.

Neuromodulator Assessment and Treatment for the Upper Face: An Update

Vince Bertucci, MD, FRCPC[a,b,*], Christina Huang, MD[a,1]

KEYWORDS

- Botulinum toxin • Neuromodulator • Upper face assessment • Eyebrow position • Injection depth
- Injection pattern

KEY POINTS

- When treating upper face musculature with BTX-A, it is crucial to recognize the intricate interplay between the various facial musculature and understand how they function harmoniously to create a natural, aesthetically pleasing look.
- A detailed appreciation for the muscles of facial expression, brow position and brow shape are critical when treating the upper face.
- Assessment for treatment of the upper face should include muscle bulk, symmetry, forehead height, eyebrow position and shape, rhytid patterns, and volume changes.
- When treating the frontalis, keeping injections below the line of convergence superficial will minimize the risk of brow ptosis.
- When treating the glabella, a 5 point technique with deep injections into the procerus (midline and inferior to a horizontal line connecting the upper medial brows) and medial corrugators (at the inferomedial aspect of the hair bearing brow) and superficial injections into the lateral corrugator (between the midpupillary and limbal lines, superior to the hair bearing brow) will minimize the risk of brow ptosis.
- When treating the lateral cantus, injections should be superficial, 1cm lateral to the orbital rim.

INTRODUCTION

Facial esthetics refers to the study and practice of enhancing the appearance of the face through a variety of techniques, including surgical and non-surgical injectable treatments. The importance of facial esthetics expands both medical and social realms and can impact self-confidence, emotional well-being, and overall quality of life.[1] Medically, facial esthetics plays a central role in the treatment and correction of certain conditions, such as congenital deformities, injury-related disfigurements, and effects of natural aging. In the social realm, optimization of facial esthetics can affect physical attractiveness, facial expression, and non-verbal communication.[2]

Specifically, the upper third of the face, comprising the area from the upper eyelids to the hairline, plays a critical role in facial esthetics. Studies have shown that the periorbital area provides the greatest amount of information per area and thus is the area that is most frequently first assessed by others.[3,4] The expressions of the upper third of the face have also been identified to contribute to facial recognition, gender classification, and expression categorization.[3,5–7] The glabella and eyebrow position are central to non-verbal communication, conveying emotions such as anger, fatigue, and impatience.[8] Furthermore, muscles of the upper face are required to produce a genuine smile, otherwise known as a Duchenne smile,[9] which is important in daily

[a] Department of Medicine, University of Toronto, Toronto, Ontario, Canada; [b] Private Practice, 100-8333 Weston Road, Woodbridge, Ontario L4L 8E2, Canada
[1] Present address: 2075 Bayview Ave, Toronto, ON M4N 3M5, Canada.
* Corresponding author.
E-mail address: vince.bertucci@utoronto.ca

Dermatol Clin 42 (2024) 51–62
https://doi.org/10.1016/j.det.2023.08.012
0733-8635/24/© 2023 Elsevier Inc. All rights reserved.

interactions and social connections. Not only does the esthetics of the upper face impact how one is viewed by others, enhancing this region has also been associated with a more positive internal emotional state, increased level of personal satisfaction, and improved overall quality of life.[10–16] Given the plethora of information that can be decoded at first sight and the impact on social functioning and quality of life, it is not surprising that the upper face is an area of focus for people wishing to enhance their facial appearance.

Given the crucial importance of facial appearance, it is not surprising that minimally invasive cosmetic procedures continue to rise in popularity. According to the 2020 American Society of Plastic Surgeons Statistics Report, botulinum toxin type A (BTX-A) treatments were the most commonly performed minimally invasive procedure, with a 459% increase from 2000.[17] Moreover, BTX-A was also almost 25% more popular than soft tissue fillers, the second most popular non-invasive procedure.[17]

The history of BTX-A dates back to the 1900s, when it was first used in ophthalmology to correct strabismus by selectively weakening periocular muscles.[18,19] Since then, multiple BTX-A products have been approved by the Food and Drug Administration (FDA) for the treatment of moderate to severe glabellar lines[20,21] as well as for other esthetic indications such as forehead and lateral canthal lines.

When treating upper face musculature with BTX-A, it is crucial to recognize the intricate interplay between these structures and understand how they function harmoniously to create a natural, esthetically pleasing look. This article will outline relevant upper face anatomy, provide a detailed framework for clinical assessment, and discuss advanced BTX-A injection techniques based on recent advances.

FUNCTIONAL ANATOMY

To achieve optimal esthetic outcomes when treating the upper third of the face with BTX-A, a detailed appreciation for the muscles of facial expression is critical. Additionally, one must conceptualize the muscles of the upper third of the face as a biomechanical complex that collaboratively contributes to facial expression, as the movement of each muscle influences the other muscles. The muscles of the upper third of the face that contribute to facial expression, brow position, and brow shape include the frontalis, procerus, orbicularis oculi, depressor supercilii, and corrugator supercilii (**Fig. 1**).

Frontalis

The frontalis is a rectangularly shaped muscle underlying the forehead skin (**Fig. 2**A). It originates cranially from the tendinous galea aponeurosis and inserts caudally by interdigitating with the procerus, corrugator supercilii, depressor supercilii, and medial aspects of the orbicularis oculi.[22] The vertical orientation of frontalis muscle fibers is responsible for creating horizontal forehead lines upon contraction. Laterally, the frontalis extends to the temporal fusion line.[22] While the frontalis is commonly symmetric, there may be anatomic variation. For example, some individuals have a central aponeurosis.[23] When present, there is less wrinkling of the overlying central forehead with muscle fascicles oriented more laterally, producing a more obtuse angle of forehead lines.[24] Recently, the frontalis was shown to have bidirectional movement, with the lower 60% acting as an eyebrow elevator and the upper 40% being a hairline depressor.[25] The point at which these antagonistic movement patterns converge on the forehead has been termed the "line of convergence." It is important to note that the frontalis is the sole eyebrow elevator.

Procerus

The procerus muscle is a triangular-shaped muscle originating from the nasal bone at the root of the nose (**Fig. 2**B). It becomes more superficial as it moves superiorly and inserts into the skin of the glabella at the level of the upper margin of the eyebrows.[22] At its insertion point, its fibers interdigitate with the frontalis muscle. Contraction of the procerus muscle is responsible for depression of the medial brow as well as horizontal glabellar lines.[26]

Orbicularis Oculi

The orbicularis oculi muscle is a flat, subdermal sphincter muscle that is responsible for eyelid closure and movement (**Fig. 2**C).[27,28] It is oval in shape and surrounds the eye, with fibers running in multiple directions. This muscle can be divided into 2 subunits, orbital and palpebral. The orbital subunit is the outer portion of the muscle that surrounds the orbital rim, originating from the nasal part of the frontal bone, frontal process of the maxilla, and the medial canthal tendon.[27,28] The palpebral subunit is the inner portion of the orbicularis oculi and can further be subdivided into the pretarsal and preseptal regions.[29] The pretarsal aspect overlies the tarsal plates and contributes to involuntary blinking,[27,28] while the preseptal aspect lies between the pretarsal and orbital subunits and is responsible for voluntary eye closure.[27,28] The shape of orbicularis oculi is

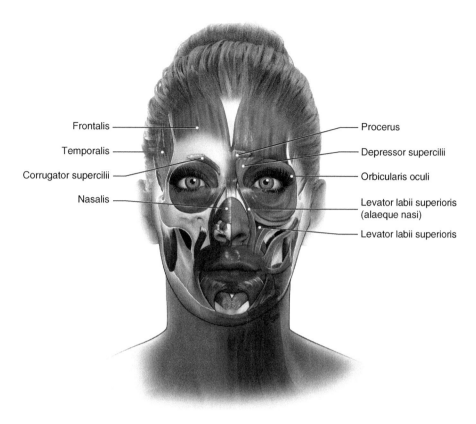

Fig. 1. Upper face muscles: The frontalis, procerus, orbicularis oculi, depressor supercilii, and corrugator supercilii muscles contribute to upper face expressions and rhytid patterns. (Tara Delle Chiaie, Essentials of Neuromodulation, 1st Edition, Academic Press, 2021.).

such that it has horizontal, vertical, and diagonal fibers, giving rise to vertical lines (superiorly and inferiorly), horizontal lines (medially and laterally), and angled lines in between, respectively.

Depressor Supercilii

The depressor supercilii muscle originates from the lateral aspect of the nasal bridge and inserts roughly 1.3 to 1.4 cm superior to the medial canthal tendon, lateral to the insertion of the corrugator supercilii (**Fig. 2**D).[29] Along with the other glabellar muscles, its contraction leads to downward pull of the eyebrows, further contributing to frowning and squinting.[22] Some consider the depressor supercilii muscle to be the medial aspect of the orbicularis oculi, rather than a separate muscle.[29]

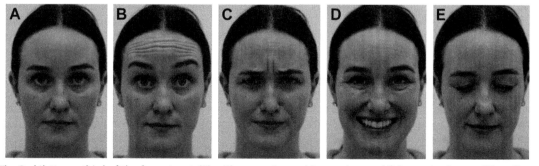

Fig. 2. (*A*) Upper third of the face at rest, (*B*) with expression: raising eyebrows, (*C*) furrowing brows, (*D*) smiling, (*E*) closing eyes tightly. Careful analysis of facial expressions and rhytid patterns is the foundation of customized treatment planning and optimal results.

Corrugator Supercilii

The corrugator supercilii muscle is a small and narrow muscle within the glabellar complex (**Fig. 2**E). It originates from the medial part of the superciliary arch of the frontal bone, sandwiched between the frontalis and orbicularis oculi muscles.[22,30] The surface landmark for its origin would be approximately 1 to 2 mm medial and inferior to the medial end of the hairy eyebrow.[30] The muscle then runs caudally and laterally as it integrates with the orbicularis oculi muscle and inserts to the underside of the dermis. Of note, as the corrugator supercilii gets more lateral, it also gets more superficial, which is an important consideration when treating this area.[31] The oblique orientation of the corrugator supercilii allows for it to pull the eyebrows down and medial, producing vertical "11" lines in the glabella.[26]

CLINICAL ASSESSMENT OF THE UPPER FACE
Initial Assessment

The foundation of optimized treatments and outstanding results lies in comprehensive facial assessment prior to BTX-A administration. This section will detail important considerations when evaluating patients for upper face BTX-A treatment, including muscle bulk, symmetry, forehead height, eyebrow position and shape, rhytid patterns, and volume changes. Understanding these components and how they function interdependently can help injectors create optimized, tailored treatment plans.

Muscle Bulk

Evaluation of muscle bulk through inspection and palpation is an important consideration as it impacts the effectiveness and outcomes of the procedure. The natural aging process results in decreased muscle bulk and muscle strength.[32] With time, there is also a gradual decrease in motor neurons, neuromuscular junctions, and available botulinum toxin receptors,[32] which can theoretically explain the lower doses of BTX-A required in some older patients to achieve the desired effect.

Sex differences can also influence muscle bulk and thus the amount of BTX-A required. In general, men have significantly more skeletal muscle mass compared to women.[33] While studies examining facial muscle mass between sexes are limited, men have been reported to have greater facial movement during lip pursing, cheek puffing, and eye-opening animations, after adjusting for face size.[34] Thus, it is not surprising that male patients may require a higher dose of BTX-A to achieve

the same endpoint as compared to their female counterparts. In support of higher doses needed for men is a 2013 study showing that typical BTX-A dosing for the forehead is 10 to 20 units for women and 20 to 30 units for men.[22]

Another important contributor to muscle bulk is muscle location, function, and distribution. Naturally thinner muscles such as the corrugators will require lower doses compared to larger and thicker muscles of mastication like the masseter.

Lastly, preceding treatments with BTX-A may result in muscle atrophy and a smaller baseline muscle bulk. Reduced muscle size means that less BTX-A will be required to achieve the same effect.

To achieve esthetically pleasing results and avoid overtreatment or undertreatment, age and gender of the patient, muscle location, prior neuromodulator treatment, and degree of muscle bulk should be considered to adequately gauge the appropriate quantity of toxin that is required.

Symmetry

Evaluation of upper face symmetry is crucial when formulating injection doses and patterns. It is important to recognize that at baseline, up to 90% of individuals have some degree of frontalis and brow asymmetry.[35] While injectors commonly treat the upper third of the face equally on both sides, a retrospective review of 845 patients found that 5% of patients required a touch-up injection for eyebrow asymmetry after frontalis treatment with symmetric injection points.[35] This suggests that neuromodulator treatment can unmask subtle underlying asymmetries and highlights the need for an individualized approach. Patients may require varying doses or slightly asymmetric product placement to address baseline asymmetry and prevent exacerbation of baseline asymmetry.

Forehead Height

Forehead height is an important consideration when treating the upper face with BTX-A, given the variability from person to person and the role of the frontalis in eyebrow position. Males tend to have a taller forehead than females, which may require more than one row of BTX-A to adequately treat the entire area.[36–38] Additionally, males have been found to have more frontalis contraction to optimize visual fields, leading to deeper and more noticeable forehead rhytids.[39] Another scenario which may require multiple rows of injection is the presence of a receding hairline, thus elongating the forehead.[40,41] As the frontalis is a highly responsive muscle, and to avoid brow ptosis, some authors recommend treating the upper forehead lines at the initial visit, and then treating any residual lower forehead lines at a subsequent visit.[39]

Conversely, it is essential to identify shorter foreheads. Because the frontalis is the sole eyebrow elevator, unintentional overtreatment of patients with a short forehead puts them at risk for eyebrow and eyelid ptosis. Recent literature describes a bimodal pattern of frontalis movement.[25] As mentioned previously, there is caudal movement of the upper forehead and cranial movement of the lower forehead, resulting in downward movement of the hairline and eyebrow elevation. The horizontal line where these 2 opposing actions meet has been termed the "line of convergence" and has been described to be located at approximately 60% of the forehead height, measured from the orbital rim.

Understanding these concepts highlights the importance of forehead height assessment when planning BTX-A dosage and injection pattern.

EYEBROW POSITION AND SHAPE

A common focus of upper face BTX-A treatment is optimization of brow shape and position, as these are key determinants of non-verbal cues and overall facial appearance.[30] Careful inspection of the interplay between brow depressors (corrugator supercilii, depressor supercilii, orbicularis oculi, and procerus) and the sole brow elevator (frontalis), at rest and in motion, is an imperative step to enhancing eyebrow position and shape.

Additionally, eyebrow ptosis is common with age[42] and should be evaluated in all patients before proceeding with upper face treatment. Failure to do so may lead to exacerbation of an underlying ptosis, or unmasking of a compensated eyelid ptosis.[22,30,43,44] Eyebrow ptosis can be detected by examining the relative height of the medial and lateral brows at rest.[45] Any evidence of a shortened brow to pupil distance, disproportionate sag in the lateral brow, brow asymmetry, or a hairy brow that lies below the orbital rim should raise suspicion for eyebrow ptosis.[42]

It is also important to differentiate between true ptosis and pseudoptosis.[45] True ptosis is defined as eyelid drooping due to muscle weakness. Pseudoptosis is thought to be caused by many factors unrelated directly to muscle weakness but by excess skin, fat, trauma, or neoplasms.[46] More subtle signs of eyebrow ptosis include prominent forehead horizontal lines, eyelid hooding, or dermatochalasis.

In addition to eyebrow ptosis, it is equally important to identify eyelid ptosis. Eyelid ptosis is commonly caused by age-related dysfunction of the levator palpebrae superioris. One study suggested that eyelid ptosis occurs in 2.5% to 11.6% of individuals aged 45 to 69 years and up to 43% of people over 70.[47] When assessing for eyelid or eyebrow ptosis, the patient should be upright, relaxed, and looking straight ahead.[45] The marginal reflex distance (distance from the corneal light reflex to the upper eyelid margin) has been proposed as a more objective measure for eyelid ptosis.[48] In non-Asians and Asians, a distance of 3.5 to 5.5 and 2.2 to 3.7 mm is considered normal, respectively. A marginal reflex distance of less than 3 indicates the presence of ptosis.[48,49]

Rhytid Patterns

Recognition of various rhytid patterns and individualized anatomy of the upper face will assist in dosing and injection pattern of BTX-A. Areas that will be highlighted in this section include the forehead, orbicularis oculi, and glabella.

Horizontal forehead lines created by the frontalis typically follow 1 of 2 patterns: a wavy or "V" pattern, or continuous horizontal pattern (**Fig. 3**).

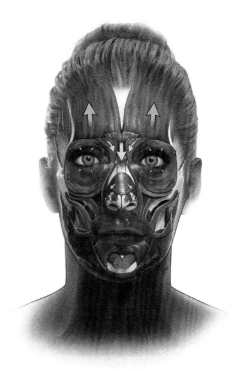

Fig. 3. Functional anatomy of the upper third of the face. Note the direction of muscle contraction for each of the upper facial muscles, which influences rhytid patterns. (Tara Delle Chiaie, Essentials of Neuromodulation, 1st Edition, Academic Press, 2021.).

This presence of a central decussation in the frontalis muscle is associated with a wavy or "V" pattern. Wider "V" patterns correlate with a wider decussation and lower neurotoxin dosing to achieve esthetically pleasing outcomes.[23]

Lateral canthal or "crow's feet" lines can follow several wrinkle patterns.[50,51] The full-fan pattern involves wrinkling from the lower lateral brow, across the upper eyelid, through the lateral canthus. The upper fan pattern involves wrinkling in the upper eyelid down to the lateral canthus. This is considered to be the least common pattern, involving less than 10% of patients.[51] The central fan pattern describes rhytids localized in the skin adjacent to the lateral canthus. Lastly, the lower fan pattern involves wrinkles in the lower eyelid and upper cheek (see **Fig. 3**). Although categorized into 4 patterns, there is significant heterogeneity and overlap in lateral canthus rhytid patterns, highlighting the importance of individualized treatment planning.[51]

Glabellar contraction patterns have been classified according to the predominance of eyebrow approximation, depression, or elevation movements.[8,16] These include the "U," "V," "converging arrows," "omega," and "inverted omega" patterns (see **Fig. 3**). Authors in Korea suggested an alternative naming system for individuals of Asian descent, including the "U," "X," "11," "Phi," and "I" patterns.[52]

Volume Changes

Comprehensive esthetic evaluation of the face must include volume loss and fat atrophy as they commonly contribute to rhytids and should be addressed in the context of neuromodulator treatment. Cadaveric studies have shown that facial subcutaneous fat is compartmentalized, with redistribution and decrease in size with age.[50] Loss of subcutaneous volume allows excess superficial skin to sag into rhytid valleys, further accentuating wrinkles. Moreover, redistribution and loss of fat in the upper face can cause underprojection of the brows, a sunken appearance to the forehead, and a concave appearance of the temples. Each of these represents signs of aging and should be addressed with procedures such as soft tissue fillers to optimize BTX-A results.

TREATMENT OF THE UPPER FACE
Patient Positioning

The importance of patient positioning during treatment cannot be overstated. Ensuring patient comfort while optimizing injector ergonomics so as to permit precise injection is the key. One group proposed that the patient be seated upright with the head supported by a headrest, at the level of the injector's shoulder.[53] The authors feel that the ideal patient position will be physician and patient dependent. Their preference is to have the patient lying back at an angle of approximately 80° with the head supported, such that the height of the area to be injected is slightly lower than the injector's head.

Product Selection and Reconstitution

There are currently 5 FDA approved formulations of BTX-A commercially available for rhytids: onabotulinumtoxin A, abobotulinumtoxin A, incobotulinumtoxin A, prabotulinumtoxin A, and daxibotulinumtoxin A. A limited number of head-to-head studies have compared the various formulations. While differences exist, all formulations are effective in treating upper facial rhytids and ultimately any product may be used.[53,54] It is important that the injector learn the clinical characteristics of their chosen product so as to achieve the desired outcome.

With regard to reconstitution, the FDA states that sterile, preservative-free 0.9% sodium chloride should be used for all approved formulations.[55–59] After reconstitution, the product should be stored between 2°C and 8°C and used within 24 hours,[55–58] except for daxibotulinutoxinA, which should be used within 72 hours.[59] These recommendations are designed to mitigate risk of infection and loss of toxin efficacy. It is important to note that reconstitution with benzyl alcohol-preserved normal saline has been shown to help reduce injection site pain without compromising potency or longevity.[54,60] Furthermore, it has also been shown that products stored at appropriate temperature can be effective for up to 6 weeks.[60–62] Some authors have suggested freezing the reconstituted product to help it retain its potency for up to 6 months.[63]

While most FDA trials utilize a standard volume of reconstition, the volume can also be tailored to the treatment site. In general, larger volumes should be used if product spread is desired, such as for the lateral canthal lines or in individuals with tall foreheads where brow ptosis is not a concern. Conversely, in areas where precision is imperative and spread to adjacent muscles may be problematic such as the glabella, smaller volumes of reconstitution may be desirable. A study in support of this concept demonstrated similar efficacy of onabotulinumtoxinA between dilutions of 100, 33.3, 20, and 10 units/mL when treating the glabella.[62] However, 6 patients developed ptosis, all of whom were treated using larger volumes of reconstitution. Thus, larger volumes for reconstitution should be avoided when spread to nearby muscles may lead to adverse effects.

Size of Needle

The product monograph for onabotulinumtoxinA recommends 30-gauge to 33-gauge needles for treatment of glabellar lines, although 30-gauge are the most frequently used.[56,63,64] While thinner needles are better tolerated from a pain perspective, they are more expensive,[64] and there have been inconsistent cost-analysis data supporting its benefits.[63–65] Many practitioners have cited their preference for the 0.3 cc U-100 insulin syringe with 31-gauge Ultra-Fine II needle due to its ease of use, cost efficiency, small size, accuracy of toxin delivery, better patient comfort, and built-in mechanisms to minimize neuromodulator loss.[66] However, no needle size has been found to be superior to another in terms of efficacy or patient comfort.

Injection Depth

The FDA label for the various neuromodulators recommends intramuscular BTX-A administration for cosmetic use. However, recent studies have reported a higher rate of brow ptosis with deeper intramuscular BTX-A injections in the forehead compared to superficial intradermal injections.[67,68] While this may indicate that depth of product placement may affect efficacy, these authors referred to their observed outcomes as adverse effects. To further correlate the effect of BTX-A depth with efficacy and forehead fascial anatomy, a prospective split-face study confirmed that injections in the supraperiosteal plane gave significantly better rhytid reduction compared to intradermal placement.[69] Furthermore, while intradermal injections decrease risks of unwanted adverse events, studies have demonstrated that superficial placement does not affect the duration of effect.[67] One downside of intradermal injection is increased pain compared to intramuscular injection.[68] With this knowledge, more superficial injections should be performed in areas where a surface effect is desired, such as on the forehead inferior to the line of convergence (**Fig. 4**). Conversely, deeper injections would be preferred when a substantial effect on the frontalis muscle is the goal, such as the forehead superior to the line of convergence.

Another site exemplifying the importance of injection depth is the glabella (**Fig. 5**). Recent evidence suggests that it is best to inject the neuromodulator deeply for the medial corrugator, and more superficially for the lateral corrugator[70] (**Fig. 6**). The aim of this technique is to avoid injecting the frontalis, which lies superficial to the medial corrugator and deep to the lateral corrugator. The corrugators originate on bone medially below the superciliary arch and as they extend laterally they become more superficial, inserting into the dermis. Furthermore, the corrugators rarely extend above the upper margin of the hair-bearing brow. Thus, the traditional injection technique in which the product is placed 1 cm above the hair-bearing brow should be avoided so as to avoid weakening the frontalis and causing brow ptosis (**Fig. 7**). Medially, injecting the inferomedial aspect of the natural

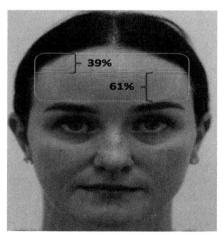 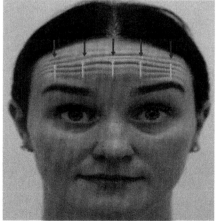

Fig. 4. Line of convergence. The line of convergence is an imaginary line located an average of approximately 60% of the distance between the brows and the hairline, and represents the line separating the upwards and downwards activity of the frontalis muscles. Superficial injections below the line will minimize the risk of brow ptosis.

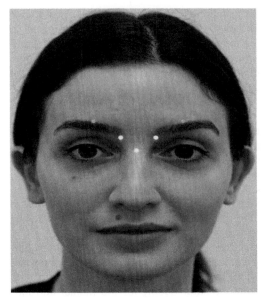

Fig. 5. Glabellar injection location and depth for glabella. Procerus: deep (yellow dots), midline, and inferior to a horizontal line connecting the upper medial brows, which is closer to the origin of the procerus muscle; medial corrugator: deep (yellow dots), at the inferomedial aspect of the hair-bearing brow, slightly medial to the medial canthal line, targeting the belly of the corrugators; lateral corrugator: superficial (blue dots), between the midpupillary and limbal lines, superior to the hair-bearing brow.

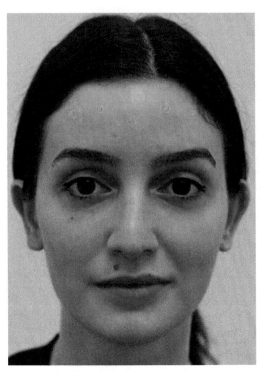

Fig. 6. Forehead injection sites. Injection sites will vary depending on forehead height, brow position, tendency to peaked brows, and superior extent of rhytids. Care must be taken to avoid brow ptosis, as described in the text. Blue dots represent sites of injection.

hair-bearing brow will best target the bulk of the medial corrugator while sparing the frontalis.

With regard to the procerus, deep injections inferior to the horizontal line connecting the medial brows, which is closer to the origin of the muscle on bone, will be most likely to weaken the procerus while sparing frontalis fibers that interdigitate with procerus. This technique is most likely to give medial brow lift and avoid brow ptosis (**Fig. 8**).

Dose and Injection Technique

As previously discussed, muscles of the upper face are closely related spatially, and as a result, treatment of one area can affect adjacent muscles and overall outcomes. Injection site in the upper face is also not one-size-fits-all. One of the main concerns when treating the glabella is inadvertent weakening of the frontalis, leading to lowering of the brows. For example, if the medial frontalis is weakened when treating the procerus, overcompensation of the lateral brow may occur leading to an unnatural quizzical or diabolical appearance.[30,44,71–73] A recent study analyzed outcomes of eyebrow position in 60 patients after glabellar treatment by 4 expert injectors using varied techniques and injection points. The most balanced brow outcomes resulted from the following injection sites[70]: (1) procerus: deep, midline, and inferior to the horizontal line connecting upper medial brows, which is closer to the origin of the procerus muscle; (2) medial corrugator: deep, at the inferomedial aspect of the hair-bearing brow, targeting the main belly of the corrugators; and (3) lateral corrugators: superficial, between the midpupil and lateral limbal lines, just superior to the hair-bearing brow. Historically, there has been hesitancy to inject BTX-A inferior to the medial brow due to a presumed risk of eyelid ptosis from neuromodulator diffusion affecting the levator palpebrae superioris.[22,74] However, the diffusion zone from the inferomedial region of the brow is relatively distant from the levator palepebrae superioris, and would thus be a lesser concern compared to the proximity of the lower frontalis muscle fibers. For the same reason, the recommended procerus injection site is more inferior than traditionally described, near the origin of the muscle, as the superior procerus interdigitates closely with the frontalis and orbicularis oculi.

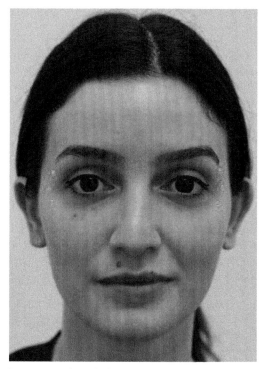

Fig. 7. Lateral canthal injection sites. Injections in this region are superficial, staying 1 cm lateral to the orbital rim. The number of injection sites may be modified based on individual patient needs.

Upper face neuromodulator dosing is highly variable, and nuances are beyond the scope of this article.

Post-Procedure Care

While there are a plethora of post-procedure care recommendations for patients receiving neuromodulators, a standard, evidence-based approach is lacking. Patients are commonly asked to exercise the injected muscles for up to 4 hours after injection to help promote cellular uptake.[75,76] While there is no evidence to support increased clinical benefit in the long term, a small study showed that exercising the treated muscles post-procedure can induce an earlier onset of effect.[76] Radiolabeling studies have shown that BTX-A binding occurs within an average of 32 to 64 minutes, suggesting that facial exercise post-treatment may only be indicated for 1 hour instead of 4 hours, as most of the binding will be complete during that time.[75,77,78] Recommendations on post-procedure restrictions are also varied and none demonstrate superior outcomes or reduced complications. Some authors recommend that patients avoid massaging their face[78] and vigorous physical exercise for 4 hours to reduce the spread of toxin to unwanted areas.[79]

The peak effect of BTX-A is typically seen by approximately 14 days. Thus, patients are seen in follow-up for reevaluation and any touch ups at this time.

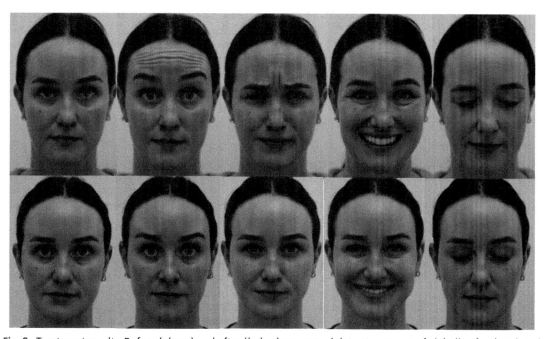

Fig. 8. Treatment results. Before (*above*) and after (*below*) neuromodulator treatment of glabellar, forehead, and lateral canthal rhytids. Note the significant rhytid reduction while maintaining brow position and natural expressions.

SUMMARY

Neuromodulator treatment of the upper face has been extensively studied and serves as an excellent tool to enhance facial appearance, nonverbal communication, and social functioning. Optimal outcomes are best achieved when health care providers take an individualized approach, based on knowledge of structural and functional anatomy, thorough facial assessment, and customized injection techniques and patterns.

CLINICS CARE POINTS

- When treating upper face musculature with BTX-A, it is crucial to recognize the intricate interplay between the various facial musculature and understand how they function harmoniously to create a natural, aesthetically pleasing look.

- A detailed appreciation for the muscles of facial expression, brow position and brow shape are critical when treating the upper face.

- Assessment for treatment of the upper face should include muscle bulk, symmetry, forehead height, eyebrow position and shape, rhytid patterns, and volume changes.

- When treating the frontalis, keeping injections below the line of convergence superficial will minimize the risk of brow ptosis.

- When treating the glabella, a 5 point technique with deep injections into the procerus (midline and inferior to a horizontal line connecting the upper medial brows) and medial corrugators (at the inferomedial aspect of the hair bearing brow) and superficial injections into the lateral corrugator (between the midpupillary and limbal lines, superior to the hair bearing brow) will minimize the risk of brow ptosis.

- When treating the lateral cantus, injections should be superficial, 1cm lateral to the orbital rim.

DISCLOSURE

None.

REFERENCES

1. Yıldız T, Selimen D. The impact of facial aesthetic and reconstructive surgeries on patients' quality of life. Indian J Surg 2015;77:831–6.
2. McKeown DJ. Impact of minimally invasive aesthetic procedures on the psychological and social dimensions of health. Plast Reconstr Surg Glob Open 2021;9(4).
3. Van Gompel RPG, Fischer MH, Murray WS, et al. Eye movements. Amsterdam: Elsevier Science; 2007.
4. Caldara R, Zhou X, Miellet S. Putting culture under the "spotlight" reveals universal information use for face recognition. PLoS One 2010;5:e9708.
5. Barton JJ, Radcliffe N, Cherkasova MV, et al. Information processing during face recognition: The effects of familiarity, inversion, and morphing on scanning fixations. Perception 2006;35:1089–105.
6. Henderson JM, Williams CC, Falk RJ. Eye movements are functional during face learning. Mem Cognit 2005;33:98–106.
7. Mäntylä T, Holm L. Gaze control and recollective experience in face recognition. Vis Cogn 2006;14:365–86.
8. De Almeida AR, da Costa Marques ER, Banegas R, et al. Glabellar contraction patterns: a tool to optimize botulinum toxin treatment. Dermatol Surg 2012;38(9):1506–15.
9. Soussignan R. Duchenne smile, emotional experience, and autonomic reactivity: a test of the facial feedback hypothesis. Emotion 2002;2(1):52.
10. Bertucci V, Almohideb M, Pon K. Approaches to Facial Wrinkles and Contouring. In: Kantor J, editor. Dermatologic Surgery. New York: McGraw-Hill Education; 2018. p. 1243–70.
11. Fagien S, Carruthers JD. A comprehensive review of patient-reported satisfaction with botulinum toxin type a for aesthetic procedures. Plast Reconstr Surg 2008;122(6):1915–25.
12. Alam Murad, Barrett KC, Hodapp RM, et al. Botulinum toxin and the facial feedback hypothesis: Can looking better make you feel happier? J Am Acad Dermatol 2008;1061–72.
13. Heckmann M, Teichmann B, Schröder U, et al. Pharmacologic denervation of frown muscles enhances baseline expression of happiness and decreases baseline expression of anger, sadness, and fear. J Am Acad Dermatol 2003;49(2):213–6.
14. Finzi E, Wasserman E. Treatment of depression with botulinum toxin A: a case series. Dermatol Surg 2006;32(5):645–50.
15. Sommer B, Zschocke I, Bergfeld D, et al. Satisfaction of patients after treatment with botulinum toxin for dynamic facial lines. Dermatol Surg 2003;29(5):456–60.
16. Lewis MB, Bowler PJ. Botulinum toxin cosmetic therapy correlates with a more positive mood. J Cosmet Dermatol 2009 Mar;8(1):24–6.
17. "Plastic Surgery Statistics." 2020. American Society of Plastic Surgeons. Available at: www.plasticsurgery.org/news/plastic-surgery-statistics. Accessed January 27, 2023.
18. Carruthers A, Carruthers J. Botulinum toxin type A: history and current cosmetic use in the upper face. InSeminars Cutan Med Surg 2001;20(2):71–84.

19. Scott AB. Botulinum toxin injection into extraocular muscles as an alternative to strabismus surgery. J Pediatr Ophthalmol Strabismus 1980;17(1):21–5.

20. Carruthers JD, Carruthers JA. Treatment of glabellar frown lines with C. botulinum-A exotoxin. The J Dermatol Surg Oncol 1992;18(1):17–21.

21. United States Food and Drug Administration. Available at: https://www.fda.gov/media/89195/download. Accessed January 27, 2023.

22. Lorenc ZP, Smith S, Nestor M, et al. Understanding the functional anatomy of the frontalis and glabellar complex for optimal aesthetic botulinum toxin type A therapy. Aesthet Plast Surg 2013;37(5):975–83.

23. Moqadam M, Frank K, Handayan C, et al. Understanding the Shape of Forehead Lines. J Drugs Dermatol JDD 2017;16(5):471–7.

24. Frank K, Freytag DL, Schenck TL, et al. Relationship between forehead motion and the shape of forehead lines—A 3D skin displacement vector analysis. J Cosmet Dermatol 2019;18(5):1224–9.

25. Cotofana S, Freytag DL, Frank K, et al. The bidirectional movement of the frontalis muscle: introducing the line of convergence and its potential clinical relevance. Plast Reconstr Surg 2020;145(5):1155–62.

26. Bentsianov B, Blitzer A. Facial anatomy. Clin Dermatol 2004;22(1):3–13.

27. Patrinely JR, Anderson RL. Anatomy of the orbicularis oculi and other facial muscles. Adv Neurol 1988;49:15.

28. Marur T, Tuna Y, Demirci S. Facial anatomy. Clin Dermatol 2014;32(1):14–23.

29. Cook BE Jr, Lucarelli MJ, Lemke BN. The depressor supercilii muscle: anatomy, histology, and cosmetic implications. The Am J Cosmet Surg 2000;17(4):193–205.

30. Cotofana S, Solish N, Gallagher C, et al. The anatomy behind eyebrow positioning: a clinical guide based on current anatomic concepts. Plast Reconstr Surg 2022;149(4):869–79.

31. Lee HJ, Lee KW, Tansatit T, et al. Three-Dimensional Territory and Depth of the Corrugator Supercilii: Application to Botulinum Neurotoxin Injection. Clin Anat 2020;33(5):795–803.

32. Nestor MS, Kleinfelder RE, Pickett A. The use of botulinum neurotoxin type A in aesthetics: key clinical postulates. Dermatol Surg 2017;43:S344–62.

33. Janssen I, Heymsfield SB, Wang Z, et al. Skeletal muscle mass and distribution in 468 men and women aged 18–88 yr. J Appl Physiol 2000. https://doi.org/10.1152/jappl.2000.89.1.81.

34. Clark Weeden J, Trotman CA, Faraway JJ. Three dimensional analysis of facial movement in normal adults: influence of sex and facial shape. The Angle Orthodontist 2001;71(2):132–40.

35. Kashkouli MB, Amani A, Jamshidian-Tehrani M, et al. Eighteen-point abobotulinum toxin a upper face rejuvenation: an eye plastic perspective on 845 subjects. Ophthalmic Plast Reconstr Surg 2014;30(3):219–24.

36. Green JB, Keaney TC. Aesthetic treatment with botulinum toxin: approaches specific to men. Dermatol Surg 2017;43:S153–6.

37. Scherer MA. Specific aspects of a combined approach to male face correction: botulinum toxin A and volumetric fillers. J Cosmet Dermatol 2016;15(4):566–74.

38. Haiun M, Cardon-Fréville L, Picard F, et al. Peculiarities of botulinum toxin injections for aesthetic treatment of the face in men. A review of the literature. Ann Aesthet Plast Surg 2019;64(3):259–65. Elsevier Masson.

39. Flynn TC. Botox in men. Dermatol Ther 2007;20(6):407–13.

40. Rossi AM. Men's Aesthet Dermatol. Semin Cutan Med Surg 2014;33(4):188–97.

41. Keaney T. Male aesthetics. Skin Ther Lett 2015;20(2):5–7.

42. Swift A, Liew S, Weinkle S, et al. The facial aging process from the "inside out". Aesthet Surg J 2021;41(10):1107–19.

43. Cotofana S, Pedraza AP, Kaufman J, et al. Respecting upper facial anatomy for treating the glabella with neuromodulators to avoid medial brow ptosis—A refined 3-point injection technique. J Cosmet Dermatol 2021;20(6):1625–33.

44. Carruthers A, Carruthers J. Eyebrow height after botulinum toxin type A to the glabella. Dermatol Surg 2007;33:S26–31.

45. Bertucci V, Carruthers JD, Sherman DD, et al. Integrative Assessment for Optimizing Aesthetic Outcomes When Treating Glabellar Lines With Botulinum Toxin Type A: An Appreciation of the Role of the Frontalis. Aesthet Surg J 2022. https://doi.org/10.1093/asj/sjac267.

46. Cohen AJ, Weinberg DA. Pseudoptosis Eval Management Blepharoptosis 2011;61–5.

47. Bacharach J, Lee WW, Harrison AR, et al. A review of acquired blepharoptosis: prevalence, diagnosis, and current treatment options. Eye 2021;35(9):2468–81.

48. Latting MW, Huggins AB, Marx DP, et al. Clinical evaluation of blepharoptosis: distinguishing age-related ptosis from masquerade conditions. InSeminars Plast Surg 2017;31(01):005–16. Thieme Medical Publishers.

49. Murchison AP, Sires BA, Jian-Amadi A. Margin reflex distance in different ethnic groups. Arch Facial Plast Surg 2009;11(5):303–5.

50. Rohrich RJ, Pessa JE. The fat compartments of the face: anatomy and clinical implications for cosmetic surgery. Foundational Pap Oculoplastics 2007;13.

51. Kane MA, Cox SE, Jones D, et al. Heterogeneity of crow's feet line patterns in clinical trial subjects. Dermatol Surg 2015;41(4):447–56.

52. Kim HS, Kim C, Cho H, et al. A study on glabellar wrinkle patterns in Koreans. J Eur Acad Dermatol Venereol 2014;28(10):1332–9.

53. Erickson BP, Lee WW, Cohen J, et al. The role of neurotoxins in the periorbital and midfacial areas. Facial Plast Surg Clin 2015;23(2):243–55.

54. Dover JS, Monheit G, Greener M, et al. Botulinum toxin in aesthetic medicine: myths and realities. Dermatol Surg 2018;44(2):249.

55. United States Food and Drug Administration. Available at: https://www.galderma.com/sites/default/files/inline-files/Dysport-aesthetic-PM-E.pdf. Accessed April 30, 2023.

56. United States Food and Drug Administration. Available at: https://www.accessdata.fda.gov/drug-satfda_docs/label/2009/103000s5109s5210lbl.pdf. Accessed April 30, 2023.

57. United States Food and Drug Administration. Available at: https://www.accessdata.fda.gov/drugsatfda_docs/label/2018/125360s073lbl.pdf. Accessed April 30, 2023.

58. United States Food and Drug Administration. https://www.accessdata.fda.gov/drugsatfda_docs/label/2019/761085s000lbl.pdf. Accessed April 30, 2023.

59. United States Food and Drug Administration. Available at: https://www.accessdata.fda.gov/drugsatfda_docs/label/2022/761127s000lbl.pdf. Accessed April 30, 2023.

60. Liu A, Carruthers A, Cohen JL, et al. Recommendations and current practices for the reconstitution and storage of botulinum toxin type A. J Am Acad Dermatol 2012;67(3):373–8.

61. Carruthers A, Carruthers J, Cohen J. Dilution volume of botulinum toxin type A for the treatment of glabellar rhytides: does it matter? Dermatol Surg 2007;33:S97–104.

62. Hui JI, Lee WW. Efficacy of fresh versus refrigerated botulinum toxin in the treatment of lateral periorbital rhytids. Ophthal Plast Reconstr Surg 2007;23(6):433–8.

63. Alam M, Geisler A, Sadhwani D, et al. Effect of needle size on pain perception in patients treated with botulinum toxin type A injections: a randomized clinical trial. JAMA Dermatol 2015;151(11):1194–9.

64. Price KM, Williams ZY, Woodward JA. Needle preference in patients receiving cosmetic botulinum toxin type A. Dermatol Surg 2010;36(1):109–12.

65. Yomtoob DE, Dewan MA, Lee MS, et al. Comparison of pain scores with 30-gauge and 32-gauge needles for periocular botulinum toxin type a injections. Ophthalmic Plast Reconstr Surg 2009;25(5):376–7.

66. Flynn TC, Carruthers A, Carruthers J. Surgical pearl: the use of the Ultra-Fine II short needle 0.3-cc insulin syringe for botulinum toxin injections. J Am Acad Dermatol 2002;46(6):931–3.

67. Jun JY, Park JH, Youn CS, et al. Intradermal injection of botulinum toxin: a safer treatment modality for forehead wrinkles. Ann Dermatol 2018;30(4):458–61.

68. Kim YJ, Lim OK, Choi WJ. Are there differences between intradermal and intramuscular injections of botulinum toxin on the forehead? Dermatol Surg 2020;46(12):e126–31.

69. Davidovic K, Melnikov DV, Frank K, et al. To click or not to click–The importance of understanding the layers of the forehead when injecting neuromodulators–A clinical, prospective, interventional, split-face study. J Cosmet Dermatol 2021;20(5):1385–92.

70. Bertucci V, Green JB, Fezza JP, et al. Impact of Glabellar Injection Technique With Daxibotulinum-toxinA for Injection on Brow Position. Aesthet Surg J 2022. sjac002.

71. Yalçınkaya E, Cingi C, Söken H, et al. Aesthetic analysis of the ideal eyebrow shape and position. Eur Arch Oto-Rhino-Laryngology 2016;273:305–10.

72. Kassir M, Gupta M, Galadari H, et al. Complications of botulinum toxin and fillers: A narrative review. J Cosmet Dermatol 2020;19(3):570–3.

73. El-Khoury JS, Jabbour SF, Awaida CJ, et al. The impact of botulinum toxin on brow height and morphology: a randomized controlled trial. Plast Reconstr Surg 2018;141(1):75–8.

74. Benedetto AV, Lahti JG. Measurement of the anatomic position of the corrugator supercilii. Dermatol Surg 2005;31(8):923–7.

75. Hsu TS, Dover JS, Kaminer MS, et al. Why make patients exercise facial muscles for 4 hours after botulinum toxin treatment? Arch Dermatol 2003;139(7):948.

76. Alam M, Geisler A, Warycha M, et al. Effect of post injection facial exercise on time of onset of botulinum toxin for glabella and forehead wrinkles: A randomized, controlled, crossover clinical trial. J Am Acad Dermatol 2019;80(4):1144–7.

77. Huang W, Foster JA, Rogachefsky AS. Pharmacology of botulinum toxin. J Am Acad Dermatol 2000;43(2):249–59.

78. Kordestani R, Small KH, Rohrich RJ. Advancements and refinement in facial neuromodulators. Plast Reconstr Surg 2016;138(4):803–6.

79. Qaqish C. Botulinum toxin use in the upper face. Atlas Oral Maxillofac Surg Clin North Am 2016;24(2):95–103.

Neurotoxin in the Lower Third of the Face

Stefania Guida, MD, PhD

KEYWORDS

• Botulinum toxin • Lower face • Chin • Masseter

KEY POINTS

- Knowledge of anatomy of the lower face is essential to understand injection sites, depth of injection, and dosage.
- Doctors should be aware of asymmetry at baseline and potential asymmetry arising after treatment and monitor after two weeks in case of correction is needed.
- Good selection of patients for inclusion and exclusion criteria and skin quality evaluation
- Consider that the aim is to reduce muscle contraction mostly and not to block muscles to reshape the face through balance muscle force

 Video content accompanies this article at http://www.derm.theclinics.com.

INTRODUCTION

Noninvasive treatments for skin rejuvenation are increasingly requested.[1–3] Botulinum toxin (BT) is the main treatment of face rejuvenation, according to statistics in the aesthetic field.[4] BT has been proven to be a safe treatment, even after repetition of sessions over several years.[5]

BT is produced by *Clostridium botulinum* and 7 of its isoforms have been described (BoNT A–G). Of these, BT-A and BT-B are commercially available for clinical applications.[6]

Both BT-A and BT-B are composed of a heavy chain, binding to the cholinergic nerve terminal, and a light chain, inhibiting the release of acetylcholine from presynaptic vesicles.[7,8] The difference between the two isoforms is the type of protein that the light chain cleaves, leading to diverse procedures in which the two BT types are used.[8,9]

Of note, apart from the inhibition of acetylcholine release, there are additional mechanisms related to BT action, such as inhibition of norepinephrine,

substance P, calcitonin gene-related peptide, and glutamate.[9] Furthermore, BT has been shown to act also on nonneuronal cells such as cells located in the skin and subcutaneous fat as well as on blood cells, therefore contributing to the wide spectrum of BT functions.[10]

Historically, in 1980s, BT has been approved by the US Food and Drug Administration for strabismus and blepharospasm treatment. After that, a progressive approval for esthetic indications for the upper face rejuvenation has been introduced since 2002.[11]

However, despite the wide number of BT-A studies for lower face treatment reported in the literature—related to onabotulinum toxin, abobotulinum toxin, and incobotulinum toxin—and the results coming from daily practice, the current application of BT for lower face treatment is still off-label.

The aim of this study is to provide an up-to-date narrative review, together with theoretical and practical tips for lower-face treatment with BT.

Funding: none.
Dermatology, Vita-Salute San Raffaele University, Via Olgettina n. 60, Milano 20132, Italy
E-mail address: guida.stefania@hsr.it

Dermatol Clin 42 (2024) 63–67
https://doi.org/10.1016/j.det.2023.06.002
0733-8635/24/© 2023 Elsevier Inc. All rights reserved.

APPLICATIONS

Lower face has been defined as the area located below the corner of the mouth,[12] therefore several indications for the lower face have been described: lip lines/wrinkles, corner of the mouth and melomental fold (marionette lines), chin area, and masseteric hypertrophy. Additionally, as the lower face is usually considered in anatomic continuity with the neck, BT treatment of the platysma and the microbotox contributes to the improvement of the lower face.

Lip Lines/Wrinkles

With passing years, vertical lines appear on the upper and lower lip areas. These lines are related to both volume loss and muscle contraction of the orbicularis oris muscle. Accordingly, even after the filler treatment of the lips, these lines can persist. BT treatment can therefore assist in the treatment of these lip lines.[12,13]

Lip lines (wrinkles) have been graded in static and dynamic conditions, according to a 5 point validated scale, that can assist clinicians and patients in assessment at baseline and in the evaluation of changes after treatment.[14]

Basically, 2 techniques for BT treatment of the lips can be considered. First of all, to treat mild and severe lip wrinkles, it has been suggested to inject BT 2 to 5 mm from the vermillion border with 2 injections per side for upper lips and one injection point per side for lower lips, for a total of 4 to 12 U.[13,15]

Additionally, to improve lip fullness appearance, it has also been suggested to inject BT at the vermillion border.[13]

Corner of the Mouth and Melomental Fold

Melomental folds or marionette lines are characterized by the downward appearance of the corner of the mouth, provoking a sad and unpleasant look, related to both the ptosis of the cheeks, with the contribution of hypertonia of the depressor anguli oris (DAO) muscle. Therefore, this area can be either correct with fillers or approached with BT. The DAO muscle acts in opposition to the zygomaticus major and minor, to promote muscle balance.[13] The site of BT injection is located 1 cm laterally the labiomental fold and above the lower mandibular margin (**Fig. 1**).[12,16] A dose of 2 to 8 U onabotulinumtoxin A or 10 to 20 s U is recommended, with 5 to 10 s U abobotulinum per point.[15] injected with up to one-half needle depth with an angle of 90° is recommended.[12]

It is important to perform an appropriate treatment considering both the point of injection as well as avoiding hyperdilution of BT to avoid the spread of product. In fact, apart from possible adverse local reactions or asymmetry after treatment, other complications might occur. For instance, if the injection is performed too medially, it can weaken the depressor labii and flattening of the lower lip contour while attempting to pronounce an "O," while if it is too high, it can impair speech and suction interfering with the orbicularis oris muscle function.

Chin area

Dimpling chin (golf-ball or peau d'orange) may be related to hypertonia of the mentalis muscle. In fact, mentalis muscle is characterized by muscle fibers oriented vertically from the bone to the skin, determining chin soft tissue and lower lip elevation, enhancing the mental crease appearance (Video 1).[12] On the basis of the results of expert consensus, an overall dose of 3 to 24 U of BT should be used with a single or double point of treatment, depending on the width of the chin, located 1 cm above the lower margin of the chin and at least 1.5 cm away from the lower lip. Needle depth can vary from half to full.[12,16] Once a double-site of injection has been chosen, each point should be located 5 mm from the midline (see **Fig. 1**).[13]

Masseteric Hypertrophy

The masseter muscle has the function to elevate the mandible and it is important in chewing activity. However, the continuous clenching of the jaw or bruxism contribute to muscle enlargement with consequent hypertrophy.[12] Masseteric

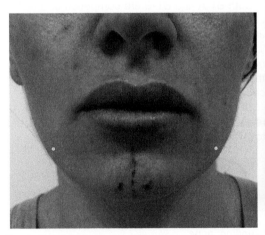

Fig. 1. Frontal picture showing the lower face of a 38 year old woman. Black circles show injection sites for the mentalis while green circles mark depressor anguli oris injection sites.

hypertrophy may be related to both esthetic and functional issues, therefore leading to BT treatment request.

To easily identify the muscle, it is possible to make the patient clench teeth.[16] A safety zone of the muscle can be identified being located below the line connecting the ear lobe and the corner of the mouth and between the posterior margin of the muscle and 1 cm posterior to the anterior palpable border of the mouth.[17] Operating within this area, recommendations suggest most commonly 3 points of injection, using a total amount of 24 to 60 U of onabotulinum toxin or incobotulinum toxin and 60 to 300 U of abobotulinum toxin A with a 30 G needle deep to the muscle.[12,16–19]

Higher dosages are usually indicated in Asians. The injection sites can be identified above the mandible angle and 2 points 1 cm lateral to the anterior margin of the masseter muscle (**Fig. 2**).[12,17] Treatment effectiveness on volume muscle reduction has been reported 3 months after treatment; furthermore, sessions can be repeated after 6 months.

Platysma Bands/Jawline

Platysma muscle has an important role in sustaining the weight of the head anteriorly and contributes to the shape of the lower face.[12]

This muscle can be treated in the area of the jawline with 6 points in the lateral area of the lower face/upper neck (upper portion of the muscle) for

an overall amount of 12 to 24 U of BT with one-third needle depth.[12]

Interestingly, the lower portion of the platysma muscle runs down the lateral neck and inserts into the fascia pectoralis.[12] The hypercontraction of this area results in platysmal bands appearance. Different approaches to platysmal bands have been described including 3 injections sites in the medial ones and 4 into the lateral ones, each band with a dose of 2 U of onabotulinum toxin, for a total of up to 28 U. One-third of needle length should be used, while pinching the band with the contralateral hand, to help performing the procedure.

To exclude patients with inadequate skin tone is pivotal for achieving the expected results and not increasing skin laxity evidence.[20]

Other Applications of Botulinum Toxin in Lower Face

Interestingly, microbotox is a recent technique consisting in injecting small aliquotes of BT into the dermal layer to improve skin quality through action on the dermal adnexa, while still obtaining a mild effect on the deeper mimic muscles through diffusion.

Specifically, a recent review revealed that heterogeneous protocols have been applied, including dilutions of BT from 2 to 10 times higher than those described on the summary of product characteristics. Microbotox has been performed with all BT types including abobotulinum, onabotulinum, and incobotulinum toxin. Results achieved with microbotox according to this review were mid-lower face-lifting and fine wrinkles reduction in cheeks especially in younger-aged subjects. Additionally, neck rejuvenation and recontouring of lower mandibular border have been found to be improved.[21,22]

Specifically, an improvement in cervicomental angle, elevation of the jowls, reduction of horizontal skin creases and vertical platysmal banding, and an improved texture of the overlying skin have been observed.[12]

Combined noninvasive treatments for the lower third of the face include fillers (**Fig. 3**), microfocused ultrasound, and threads.[1,3,23]

PRACTICAL TIPS FOR BOTULINUM TOXIN USE ON THE LOWER FACE

BT use on the lower third of the face encompasses different dilutions, depth of injection, and dosage of BT as compared with the upper face. Importantly, a specific knowledge of the anatomy of the area and selection of patients is pivotal to achieve good results.[24]

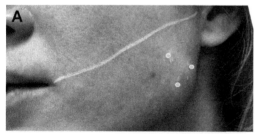

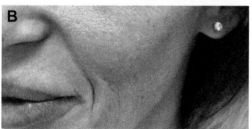

Fig. 2. Lateral pictures showing the lower face of 43 year old woman with bruxism, (*A*) patients clenching teeth to identify 3 injection sites, marked in green (before treatment) and (*B*) result after botulinum toxin treatment (3 months after treatment).

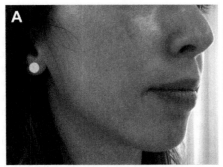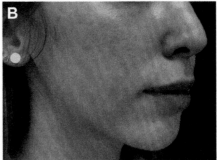

Fig. 3. Young patient with hypercontraction of the mentalis muscle (*A*) before treatment (*B*) after combined treatment with botulinum toxin and 1 ml of filler.

In addition, the aim of BT on the lower face should be to relax muscle and not to block. Therefore, using low doses of BT with higher concentration should be considered to avoid adverse events related to potential diffusion. This approach enables to target the correct area and restor muscle balance. Furthermore, more superficial injections may reduce the occurrence of adverse events. Assessment at baseline in both static and dynamic conditions can be performed according to validated scales.[14]

This is of capital importance to highlight eventual asymmetries and plan the BT accordingly (Supplementary Video 1), considering the patients' expectations and need.[12]

CONTRAINDICATIONS AND SIDE EFFECTS

Contraindications of BT are those included in the summary of product characteristics of each BT-A type and overlap those considered for the upper-face treatment, such as neuromuscular disease, pregnancy, and hypersensitivity to the drug.

Side effects of BT injections include local reactions at the site of injection such as transient swelling or bruising, asymmetries, mild headache, and flulike symptoms.[25,26]

SUMMARY

BT is the most required treatment of upper-face rejuvenation. However, recently, the application of BT on the lower face has enabled to create balance in muscle strength to smooth and lift. Indication for treatment and tips to be followed have been summarized in this study and should be considered to be able to achieve good results and avoid complications. A good selection of patients and accurate assessment are the first aspects to consider. Knowledge of anatomy of the lower face and neck and appropriate dosage, concentration, and depth of injection of BT are mandatory to treat lower third of the face with BT.

CLINICS CARE POINTS

- Botulinum toxin used in the lower third of the face is an off-label application.
- BT treatment of lower face requires knowledge of the anatomy, techniques and tips for the procedure.

DISCLOSURE

None.

SUPPLEMENTARY DATA

Supplementary data related to this article can be found online at https://doi.org/10.1016/j.det.2023.06.002.

REFERENCES

1. Guida S, Persechino F, Rubino G, et al. Improving mandibular contour: A pilot study for indication of PPLA traction thread use. J Cosmet Laser Ther 2018;20:465–9.
2. Guida S, Pellacani G, Bencini PL. Picosecond laser treatment of atrophic and hypertrophic surgical scars: In vivo monitoring of results by means of 3D imaging and reflectance confocal microscopy. Skin Res Technol 2019;25:896–902. Epub 2019 Jul 23. PMID: 31338926.
3. Rovatti PP, Pellacani G, Guida S. Hyperdiluted Calcium Hydroxylapatite 1: 2 for Mid and Lower Facial Skin Rejuvenation: Efficacy and Safety. Dermatol Surg 2020;46:e112–7.
4. American Society of Plastic Surgeons. ASPS National Clearinghouse of Plastic Surgery Procedural Statistics 2020. Available at: https://www.plasticsurgery.org/documents/News/Statistics/2020/plastic-surgery-statistics-full-report-2020.pdf Accessed 27th March 2023.

5. Hexsel D, Dal'Forno T, Hexsel C, et al. Long-Term Cumulative Effects of Repeated Botulinum Toxin Type A Injections on Brow Position. Dermatol Surg 2020;46:1252–4.

6. Parish JL. Commercial preparations and handling of botulinum toxin type A and type B. Clin Dermatol 2003;21(6):481–4. PMID: 14759580.

7. Endly DC, Miller RA. Oily Skin: a review of treatment options. J Clin Aesthet Dermatol 2017;10:49–55.

8. Dressler D, Saberi FA, Barbosa ER. Botulinum toxin: mechanisms of action. Arq Neuropsiquiatr 2005; 63(1):180–5. Epub 2005 Apr 13. PMID: 15830090.

9. Campanati A, Martina E, Giuliodori K, et al. Botulinum toxin off-label use in dermatology: a review. Skin Appendage Disord 2017;3(1):39–56.

10. Grando SA, Zachary CB. The non-neuronal and non-muscular effects of botulinum toxin: an opportunity for a deadly molecule to treat disease in the skin and beyond. Br J Dermatol 2018;178(5):1011–9. Epub 2018 Mar 25. PMID: 29086923.

11. Nestor MS, Han H, Gade A, et al. Botulinum toxin-induced blepharoptosis: Anatomy, etiology, prevention, and therapeutic options. J Cosmet Dermatol 2021;20(10):3133–46.

12. de Maio M, Wu WTL, Goodman GJ, et al. Alliance for the Future of Aesthetics Consensus Committee. Facial Assessment and Injection Guide for Botulinum Toxin and Injectable Hyaluronic Acid Fillers: Focus on the Lower Face. Plast Reconstr Surg 2017;140(3):393e–404e.

13. Atamoros FP. Botulinum toxin in the lower one third of the face. Clin Dermatol 2003;21(6):505–12.

14. Narins RS, Carruthers J, Flynn TC, et al. Validated assessment scales for the lower face. Dermatol Surg 2012;38(2 Spec No):333–42.

15. Ascher B, Talarico S, Cassuto D, et al. International consensus recommendations on the aesthetic usage of botulinum toxin type A (Speywood Unit)– Part II: Wrinkles on the middle and lower face, neck and chest. J Eur Acad Dermatol Venereol 2010;24(11):1285–95.

16. Signorini M, Piero Fundarò S, Bertossi D, et al. OnabotulinumtoxinA from lines to facial reshaping: A new Italian consensus report. J Cosmet Dermatol 2022;21(2):550–63.

17. Almukhtar RM, Fabi SG. The Masseter Muscle and Its Role in Facial Contouring, Aging, and Quality of Life: A Literature Review. Plast Reconstr Surg 2019;143(1):39e–48e. PMID: 30303926.

18. Shome D, Vadera S, Shiva Ram M, et al. Efficacy of Incobotulinum toxin-A for the treatment of masseter muscle hypertrophy in Asian Indian patients: A 2-year follow-up study. J Cosmet Dermatol 2020 Aug;19(8):1892–9.

19. Kundu N, Kothari R, Shah N, et al. Efficacy of botulinum toxin in masseter muscle hypertrophy for lower face contouring. J Cosmet Dermatol 2022;21(5): 1849–56.

20. Sugrue CM, Kelly JL, McInerney N. Botulinum Toxin Treatment for Mild to Moderate Platysma Bands: A Systematic Review of Efficacy, Safety, and Injection Technique. Aesthet Surg J 2019;39(2):201–6.

21. Iranmanesh B, Khalili M, Mohammadi S, et al. Employing microbotox technique for facial rejuvenation and face-lift. J Cosmet Dermatol 2022;21(10): 4160–70.

22. Galadari H, Galadari I, Smit R, et al. Use of AbobotulinumtoxinA for Cosmetic Treatments in the Neck, and Middle and Lower Areas of the Face: A Systematic Review. Toxins 2021;13(2):169.

23. Casabona G, Kaye K. Facial Skin Tightening With Microfocused Ultrasound and Dermal Fillers: Considerations for Patient Selection and Outcomes. J Drugs Dermatol 2019;18(11):1075–82. PMID: 31738490.

24. Auada Souto MP, Souto LRM. An unusual adverse event of botulinum toxin injection in the lower face. J Cosmet Dermatol 2021;20(5):1381–4.

25. Klein AW. Complications, adverse reactions, and insights with the use of botulinum toxin. Dermatol Surg 2003;29:549–56.

26. Kassir M, Gupta M, Galadari H, et al. Complications of botulinum toxin and fillers: A narrative review. J Cosmet Dermatol 2020;19(3):570–3.

The Needle Versus Cannula Debate in Soft Tissue Augmentation

Jana Al-Hage, MD[a], Hassan I. Galadari, MD[b],*

KEYWORDS

• Injectables • Fillers • Hyaluronic acid • Cannula • Needle

KEY POINTS

- Hypodermic needles have long existed before the invention of cannulas.
- Cannulas are considered safer than needles, with less risk of injury.
- Cannulas are preferred for uniformly filling large areas such as the cheeks and the jawline and for deep volumizing injections with less risk for the material to diffuse in upper vertical planes.
- Needles are preferred for small touch-ups in delicate areas such as the lips and the tear troughs.
- Both needles and cannulas are still widely used, and no one technique is the only correct choice for any application.

INTRODUCTION

Filler injections are a common practice in cosmetic dermatology and have increased in popularity because of enhanced safety profile and improved physical characteristics.[1]

Hyaluronic acid (HA) remains the most widely used filler material today across the globe, combining safety, reliability, and a relatively long duration of action.

One of the key aspects of the injectable filler procedure is the choice of delivery device—either a needle or a cannula. Although both methods have their benefits and drawbacks, the use of needle versus cannula has been a topic of debate among cosmetic practitioners.

The choice of which to use depends on many factors including the patient's specific needs, the anatomic site, the type of injectable filler, the type of defect being treated, and the practitioner's preferences, with the objective to reach the best aesthetic outcome while being the least dangerous and avoid side effects.

In this review, the authors aim to expose the advantages and disadvantages of both fillers' delivery techniques, needles versus cannulae, in order to be able to assess and compare their safety profile and precision and to describe their use in specific anatomic sites.

HISTORY OF INJECTABLE FILLERS

Starting 2003, several filler agents have emerged and were approved by the US Food and Drug Administration for cosmetic purpose. Each filler product is defined by many variables, including cohesivity, degree of cross-linking and viscosity modulus,[2] which tailor their use to the site and technique of injection.[3]

Traditionally, the use of fillers was restricted to superficial dermal layers, to eradicate creases and folds. Later on, with the concept of facial recontouring and correction of volume loss, the delivery of these fillers rapidly became performed to deeper cutaneous layers, reaching the supra-periosteal plane.[4,5] However, with the widespread

Funding sources: none.
[a] Department of Dermatology, Saint Louis Hospital, AP-HP, Groupe Hospitalier, Paris, France; [b] College of Medicine and Health Sciences, United Arab Emirates University, Al Ain, United Arab Emirates
* Corresponding author.
E-mail address: hgaladari@gmail.com

Dermatol Clin 42 (2024) 69–77
https://doi.org/10.1016/j.det.2023.06.010

derm.theclinics.com

use of these deeper injections, there was an increased report of tissue injury, with one of the most feared concern being penetrating a vessel with the sharp needle and intraarterial filler deposition.

Therefore, "needless injections" were developed and blunt tip microcannulas started to be available in around 2010—almost 30 years after the beginnings of facial fillers in cosmetic practice—with the idea that these tools were less likely to cause microvasculature laceration and vascular occlusion.[6]

However, both techniques, needles and cannulae, are still widely used for filler injections, and many of the dermal filler products nowadays are sold packaged in a syringe of 1 mL, with both a needle and a cannula allowing the practitioner to choose between the 2 options.

DEFINITION OF NEEDLES AND CANNULAE
Needle

A hypodermic needle is a thin, sharp device, usually made of stainless steel. It is disposable and available in various sizes (short vs long) and diameters (measured in gauges [G]). Those parameters are chosen based on the viscosity of the filler product and the area to be treated. Often, a needle between 27 and 31 G is used, with the length ranging between 4 and 40 mm.

Cannula

A cannula is a tunneled tip usually made of soft plastic that is flexible and has a blunt nonperforating end. Its parameters are also the diameter and length, with the most frequently used cannulas in facial injectables ranging between 25 and 32 G. They are usually available as 30-, 40-, or 50-mm length disposable and autoclavable models.[6]

ADVANTAGES OF NEEDLES
Ease of Use

Needles existed way long before cannulas were invented (**Fig. 1**). They can easily penetrate the skin because of their sharp tip and can be rapidly advanced into the tissue while visualizing its path within the tissue. There is good control over the amount injected, and larger volume of filler can be delivered in a single pass.

Precision

Needles have long been considered more precise, as the injector can exactly target the tip of the needle to the desired place ensuring accurate placement of the filler material. However, recent cadavers' experiments compared quantitively the precision of both techniques, needle versus cannulae, by using dye material or fluoroscopic imaging,[7–10] and showed that the injected product

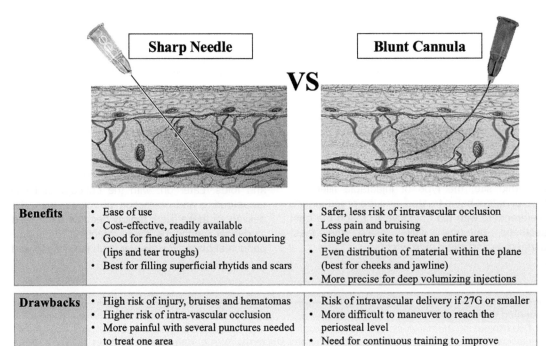

	Sharp Needle	Blunt Cannula
Benefits	• Ease of use • Cost-effective, readily available • Good for fine adjustments and contouring (lips and tear troughs) • Best for filling superficial rhytids and scars	• Safer, less risk of intravascular occlusion • Less pain and bruising • Single entry site to treat an entire area • Even distribution of material within the plane (best for cheeks and jawline) • More precise for deep volumizing injections
Drawbacks	• High risk of injury, bruises and hematomas • Higher risk of intra-vascular occlusion • More painful with several punctures needed to treat one area • Risk of diffusion of the filler into more superficial layers	• Risk of intravascular delivery if 27G or smaller • More difficult to maneuver to reach the periosteal level • Need for continuous training to improve technical skills

Fig. 1. Comparison between needles and cannulas.

may run retrograde along the perpendicular tract into more superficial layers after injections with a needle into supraperiosteal plane. Thus, filler location delivered by sharp needles may not be as precise as it had been assumed previously.

Simple Procedure for Small Areas

Needles can be considered a good choice for small or delicate areas, such as the lips and around the eyes, or to fill a targeted skin defect such as acne scars and tethered surgical depressions; this was further confirmed by the significantly reduced horizontal diffusion detected in the cadaver skins when injecting with a needle.[7]

Combining Filling with the Subcision Technique

The needle can additionally be used to transect deep stiff attachments, by applying a fanning movement or a back-and-forth movement.[7]

However, a recent review demonstrated that a modified subcision done with a blunt cannula usually of 18 G was more efficient and comfortable than when the subcision was done with a standard 27 G needle.[11,12]

Cost-Effectiveness

Needles are more widely available than cannulas, especially in underserved areas.

DISADVANTAGES OF NEEDLES

There are several drawbacks to the needle use, in particular patients may feel discomfort or pain, especially that several punctures are needed to treat an entire area (see **Fig. 1**).

Another important concern is the higher risk for microvasculature laceration, bruises, and hematomas. However, some practical techniques can help decrease this risk, for example, by adding 0.2 to 0.3 mL of 1% lidocaine with epinephrine and by aspirating for 5 seconds before injecting within a desired place.[13] However, this preventative technique is inconsistent, with the aspiration being possible only in half of the times with the needle provided with the package, especially if the filler material is too viscous, giving a false sense of security.[13,14]

ADVANTAGES OF CANNULAS
Less Traumatic

Blunt tip cannulas are less traumatic than the needles: they are flexible with less risk of tissue laceration and bruising (see **Fig. 1**). They are also longer, avoiding multiple punctures, with the ability to inject an entire nasolabial fold or lip using one single entry site. They were thus proved to decrease pain, edema, hematoma, and essentially postprocedure downtime.[15]

Easy to Deliver the Filler Material

Cannulas are usually larger than needles, thus may deliver high viscosity materials and may be easy to inject with less plunger pressure. The filler product is normally injected while moving the cannula, usually in a retrograde manner or less often with an antegrade flow.

Ability to Redirect Path Within the Tissue

Cannulas are introduced obliquely at an angle through a hole created by a larger needle (18 G needle), then moved in the supraperiosteal plane or deep subcutaneous plane in a back-and-forth motion or a rotation movement until reaching the desired level. The aesthetic practitioner may be able to feel the resistance of the structures through which a microcannula passes and can adjust the applied pressure and the angle accordingly. He can also lift the cannula after insertion to check its position: if it is within the subcutaneous space it can be easily detected through the skin but not if within the intramuscular layer.[16]

Minimize the Risk of Intravascular Injections

One of the most important aspects of cannulas is that they are less likely to penetrate important structures in the tissue, which reduces the risk of infection, hematoma, nerve damage, and vascular occlusion.[7,8]

However, studies have shown that when using a cannula of 27 G or smaller, the sharpness is almost equal to that of a needle with a similar risk of intraarterial delivery of fillers.[17,18] This risk further increases when a cannula reaches a vascular wall in a perpendicular angle. Another cadaver experiment also showed that only the 18-G and 22-G cannulas were unable to penetrate the vessel wall in facial arteries.[18]

Good Alternative for Patients with Needle Phobia

For patients presenting with needle phobia, explaining the advantages of using a cannula with much less punctures needed seems to have a positive psychological influence on the recovery.

Precision

As mentioned earlier, recent experimental studies demonstrated that the injected material remaining in its desired plane was significantly higher when using a cannula.[7,8] Therefore, cannula technique is now considered more precise than needles for deep-layer placement of fillers, as there is less risk for the material to diffuse in upper vertical planes.[19]

Homogenous Filling of Large Areas

One of the main benefits of cannulae is also the possibility to inject smoothly and uniformly over a large surface without creating bumps. In addition, experimental studies showed that the material can distribute more evenly horizontally within the same plane[7]; this makes cannulas a privileged tool when treating a large area of volume loss such as the cheeks and the jawline.

DISADVANTAGES OF CANNULAS

Cannulas are relatively new to the market. Their use requires some expertise and continuing training for the injector to acquire skills, as they are more difficult to maneuver to reach the periosteal level (see **Fig. 1**).[8] Cannulas are considered less precise when treating a delicate or targeted area, as the material can diffuse horizontally, with a risk of overfilling due to their larger size.[7]

In addition, several passes are sometimes needed to achieve the desired result.

ADVERSE EVENTS WITH BOTH NEEDLE AND/OR CANNULA

With the ever-increasing popularity of facial fillers arise more commonly adverse outcomes.[20] These outcomes range from pain, bruising, hematoma, disfiguration, and granulomatous inflammatory reaction, to more serious side effects such as vascular occlusion, necrosis, and blindness.[21,22] However, these side effects remain very rare and are usually mild and transient.

Rate of Unwanted Vascular Occlusions

The facial arterial system represents a danger zone for filler injections, and the delivery of the skin filler into a vessel by mistake may result in arterial blood flow occlusion. A large retrospective cohort demonstrated that this risk was reduced by 77% with the use of a cannula and depends on the experience of the injector. However, overall, the risk of intravascular occlusion remains extremely rare regardless of the filler type or the use of a needle or a cannula.[23]

The consequences of intravascular occlusion may be immediate skin blanching and sharp pain that may evolve into skin necrosis, scar, and ocular injury or blindness. The vascular entry point can occur mainly when injecting at the level of the supraorbital, supratrochlear, angular, and dorsal nasal arteries, especially from injections done in the glabella, nasal region, medial midface, nasolabial folds, and forehead.[24] The risk of vascular occlusion was found to be higher when injecting the lips and nasolabial folds (NLF) but was most severe when injecting the glabella.[23] Thus, the use of a cannula rather than needle is encouraged in these areas, especially early on in a career.

One of the factors to consider when injecting in a high-risk area is the size of the needle used. It is thought that a large needle is less likely to penetrate a vessel, but in the event that it does, a large bolus is rapidly delivered in a retrograde manner, thus carrying a higher risk of blindness.[25,26] On the other side, a small needle can readily penetrate a vessel, but the filler is injected slowly within the vessel, causing less serious events.

Moreover, studies have shown that in order to avoid devastating vascular occlusion and blindness when injecting in this site, the aliquot must be delivered in a very slow manner and must not exceed 0.1 mL with every pass, which is a safe volume, as it does not meet the entire supratrochlear trajectory dimensions reaching posteriorly the orbital apex.[27,28]

However, the most important thing is a thorough knowledge of the facial anatomy and to know how to quickly manage those complications, in particular with the use of hyaluronidase injections.[29]

NEEDLE VERSUS CANNULA IN SPECIAL ANATOMIC SITES

As described earlier in this review, the practice in facial injectables has shifted from only filling superficially lines and rhytids, to having a deep volumetric approach targeting specific facial sites.[30] For every zone of the face, several injection techniques have been described either with a cannula or a needle, and no one technique is the only correct choice for any application.

Forehead

To correct frontal concavity, injections should be done deep in the subperiosteal space (**Fig. 2**A).

The needle technique consists of injecting the forehead using a 90° angle and touching the bone, then deliver small boluses or retrograde linear threads without exceeding 0.025 mL per pass.[28,31] The choice of the needle size is controversial, as a 30 G needle carries a high risk of intravascular injection, but larger needles have a risk of backflow of the filler material into more superficial layers.[7]

In the cannula technique, the cannula is introduced at an oblique angle from the temporal crest and into the deeper layers of the skin with a

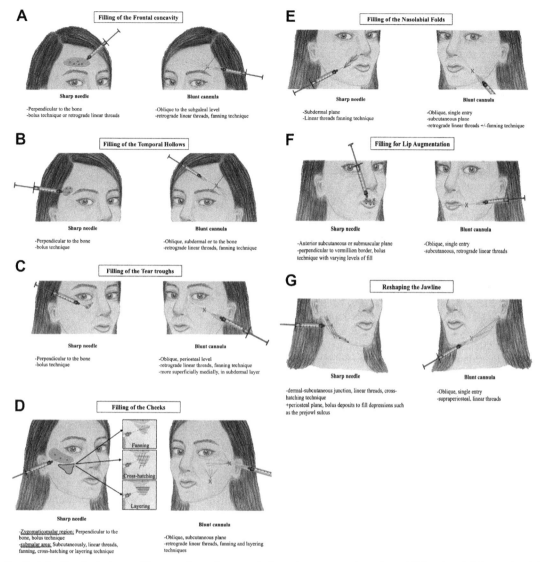

Fig. 2. Injection technique with a needle and a cannula in various anatomic regions: (A) forehead; (B) temples; (C) tear troughs; (D) cheeks; (E) nasolabial folds; (F) lips; (G) jawline.

rotating technique until it passes the resistance of the galea to reach the subgaleal level.[32] Small boluses are then injected within this plane, in a retrograde fanning technique and lightly massaged after.

Van Loghem and colleagues compared the results of both injection techniques in a split-face approach on cadavers and demonstrated that with a cannula the product was more evenly distributed and did not diffuse vertically, but with a needle there was an incident of intra-arterial injection of the lateral branch of the supraorbital artery.[8]

Therefore, a consensus member with expert opinion recommend that only blunt tip cannulas,

at least 22 G, should be used for forehead augmentation, with 0.025 to 0.04 mL per thread, bevel directed toward the periosteum.[30]

Temples

The temples are considered a high-risk area where the superficial temporal artery runs and anastomoses with the supraorbital and supratrochlear arteries, thus increasing the risk of blindness in case of embolization (Fig. 2B).[31]

The needle technique consists of injecting perpendicularly using a 27- to 30-G needle until reaching deep to the bone, then 1 to 2 microboluses are placed deep in the subcutaneous space or the superficial temporalis fascia to fill the temporal hollow.[32] It is considered safe, because even if the needle penetrates an artery, it usually traverses it through and through before reaching the desired periosteal plane.[4] However, there might be backflow diffusion of the product as explained earlier.[7]

The cannula technique consists of inserting a 22- to 25-G cannula using a temporal crest entry point, either within the subdermal space or through the fascia into the submuscular space until it reaches the periosteum, then injecting slowly small retrograde linear threads using a fanning technique, reaching a total maximum of 0.5 to 1 mL per side, followed by light massage.[28,30]

Lower Eyelids

The needle technique consists of going perpendicularly and placing multiple small blebs supraperiosteally, then mold it mechanically to spread it (**Fig. 2**C). Or one can inject with the needle tiny amounts of linear threads within the suborbicularis plane, but this carries a high risk of ecchymosis.[33]

The advantage of the needle use is that the injector can appreciate that the injections are done within the visible depression and not below it, which may result in a bulge on the upper malar area.

However, there are drawbacks to this technique: some material might diffuse to superficial layers, which may explain the risk of malar edema with HA fillers.[10,28] There might also be a high risk of ecchymosis, especially when correcting the lid-cheek demarcation laterally, as the midportion of the lid has several superficial blood vessels that can coincide with the zone of depression to correct and thus cannot be avoided. In addition, the major risk here is to inject within the angular artery that is near the medial canthus at the apex of the tear trough.

The technique with a 22- to 25-G cannula is to inject through an opening lateral to the skin insertion of the zygomatico-cutaneous ligament and advanced through the superficial muscle aponeurotic system (SMAS) to reach the periosteal level below the circular orbicularis retaining ligament. The goal is to lift the area while avoiding malar edema. Filler can be deposited in small retrograde linear threads in a fanning pattern. Finally, one can use a smaller microcannula to go medially until the cannula hits the bone ligament attachment, then the cannula is advanced more superficially in the subdermal layer to reach the medial part of the tear trough, with a total of maximum 0.1 to 0.5 mL injected per side in anterograde thread, avoiding cannulation of the angular vein.[8]

Cheeks

With the needle, fillers are injected mainly in the zygomatic-malar complex and sweeping slightly laterally and superiorly to redefine and restore the width of the midface with modest enhancement of the anterior projection (**Fig. 2**D). There are several methods of injections with a needle[33]:

One of them is by placing the product into 2 to 3 boluses deep under the malar fat pad or in the supraperiosteal plane and along the zygomatic arch, followed by molding and massage to reach the final desired shape. Another method is to place small columns injected retrogradely, while keeping in a deep plane. When submalar hollowing is severe, fillers can be lightly injected in small amounts in the subcutaneous plane using the needle in a fanning or cross-hatched fanning approach, together with the layering technique, filling deep to superficial, reaching just a neutral surface without producing a convexity.[4] The disadvantage is that there might be more noticeable needle marks on the skin, and there might be uneven spread of the filler material.

On the other hand, cannulas are used frequently to fill this area, as delivery of the material can be done more evenly and homogenously along the same horizontal plane, as demonstrated in the cadaver experiments.[7,8] A consensus advises the use of a microcannula of 30 to 40 mm when filling the medial cheek in the subcutaneous plane to minimize the risk of angular artery puncture.[30] The technique of layering, deep to superficial, is also frequently used here. Thus, fillers can be injected within the deep subcutaneous plane in a fanning technique, then within the deep dermal and subdermal space with a suggested cross-hatching strut work technique, as there is no bony support.[4]

Nasolabial Folds

Correction of this region should address both the depth of the fold and the dermal rhytids (**Fig. 2**E).

To fill the fold, ideally a fanning technique is used, with a needle inserted at the inferior aspect of the fold then advancing within the subdermal rather than intradermal plane to reach its apex to the base of the nose. Injection is done in a retrograde manner.[33] However, some practitioners prefer to best start at the superior level of the NLF, then move inferiorly, to avoid angling the needle upward and minimize the risk of intravascular injection of the angular branch of the facial artery.[4]

If there is associated moderate skin redundancy on the upper side of the NLF, a cross-hatching technique can be used transversally, with the needle inserted laterally across the fold toward the midline, with retrograde injection within the deep dermis plane or at the dermal subcutaneous junction and in very thin layers to better flatten the skin surface.

Cannula use in the NLF has been among the first applications of cannulas and is still best indicated for this region.[6,34] The risk of embolization of the angular branch of the facial artery is significantly reduced. A cannula of 22 to 25 G can be used, with a single puncture made in the inferior portion of the fold, then the cannula is introduced within the subcutaneous plane with the ability to fill the entire NLF with one single entry.[4]

Lips

The use of a needle was demonstrated to be safe and precise in this region (**Fig. 2**F). To define the natural curvatures, experts were divided on whether to use a cannula or a 30-G needle for the upper lip vermillion border.[4]

The needle technique consists of doing injections regularly and lightly along the white roll.[33] A small bleb can be deposited over the cupid's bow peak to accent these features nicely.

For lip augmentation, injections can be done midway across the vermillion width in the submuscular plane, while varying the level of fill across the lips, giving it a natural curved shape. Another technique was also described in a recent article that showed that the use of a short (4-mm) 30-G needle rather than the 13-mm (which is usually prepacked with HA fillers) was more adapted for lip augmentation. Because the labial arteries frequently run in the submucosal plane, between the oral mucosa and the orbicularis muscle, Walker and colleagues described a technique where injections are done through the vermillion border anteriorly, facilitating precise anterograde placement of HA in the safer subcutaneous plane, with less pressure needed to extrude the filler.[35]

In order to correct perioral fine lines and the philtrum columns and rhytids, a 30-G needle is preferred to do the blanching technique and a retrograde linear thread technique intradermally, respectively.[4]

For volumizing the lip or to give anterior projection to the anterior lip, a 25-G microcannula of 5 cm length, for example, is thought to be preferred to inject in the subcutaneous plane in a retrograde linear threads technique, the entry point being just lateral to the oral commissure.[6,36] Thus, one can treat an entire lip or half of it using a single-entry point, significantly reducing postintervention swelling and pain, with faster recovery. The advantage of the cannula is also that injections are much easier and much faster, as there is less back pressure needed on the syringe because of the larger bore of the cannula.

Jawline and Prejowl Sulcus

With injectables, one can treat the loss of definition of the mandibular and the notch that may appear between the chin and the jowl with aging (**Fig. 2**G).

With a 27-G needle, a cross-hatching technique can be used to start building the mandibular shape, by injecting vertical threads within the ramus and horizontal threads along the body with a 2-cm overlap over the angle of the mandible.[33] In addition, filling of depressions, especially in the prejowl space, is done using several techniques: either deep bolus deposits over the periosteum or injections within the deep dermal or dermal subcutaneous junction using a fanning, linear threading, or a cross-hatching technique.[33] The most common complication in this area is damage to the facial artery and vein and their branches, which may result in profound and prolonged ecchymosis. Patients should be informed about this risk when using a needle.

The nontraumatic cannula technique consists of using a 22- to 25-G cannula, inserted through an opening at the mandibular angle or the prejowl sulcus, then advanced directly to the periosteum, traversing the resistance of the SMAS and tendinous attachments of the masseter using the rotation technique.[4,8] Placement of the filler is then done in retrograde linear threads to distribute the product evenly, with minimal vertical diffusion to the muscle.[8]

SUMMARY

Filler injections continue to gain popularity in the armamentarium of cosmetic procedures. Both needles and cannulas are still widely used in almost all the areas of the face; however, their precision and safety profiles might differ.

Based on this literature review, and in concordance with the authors' view at the time of the writing of this article, cannula might be considered ideal to inject deep NLF, volumize the lips, and fill areas requiring high volumes of fillers such as the cheeks and the mandibular zone.

On the other hand, needles are still favored when the endpoint is to deliver the fillers intradermally, to fill small lines such as the forehead wrinkles and the vertical lip rhytides, or to correct tethered scars in association with a subcision movement. In addition, the needle can still help to refine targeted touch-ups, especially in delicate areas such as the lips and the tear troughs, which is difficult to attain when using a cannula; but the practitioner must keep in mind the associated risks.

Finally, it is important not to forget that filler injections are extremely technique dependent; therefore, it is essential that a practitioner must follow continued training to improve technical skills, in particular with the use of a cannula and with the continuous surge of off-label filler applications.

CLINICS CARE POINTS

- Anatomical knowledge remains the mainstay when injecting using both needles and cannulas.
- The necessity of injecting in the right plane, may dictate the form of injection. Cannulas cannot be used to inject the dermis.
- A task force from the American Society for Dermatologic Surgery has published evidence-based recommendations for preventing and treating adverse events of injectable fillers. Of note, fewer occlusion events occur with cannula.

DISCLOSURE

None to declare.

REFERENCES

1. Alam M, Tung R. Injection technique in neurotoxins and fillers: Indications, products, and outcomes. J Am Acad Dermatol 2018;79(3):423–35.
2. Akinbiyi T, Othman S, Familusi O, et al. Better results in facial rejuvenation with fillers. Plastic and Reconstructive Surgery Global Open 2020;8(10).
3. Tezel A, Fredrickson GH. The science of hyaluronic acid dermal fillers. J Cosmet Laser Ther 2008; 10(1):35–42.
4. Muhn C, Rosen N, Solish N, et al. The evolving role of hyaluronic acid fillers for facial volume restoration and contouring: a Canadian overview. Clin Cosmet Invest Dermatol 2012;147–58.
5. Carruthers JD, Glogau RG, Blitzer A. Advances in Facial Rejuvenation: Botulinum Toxin Type A, Hyaluronic Acid Dermal Fillers, and Combination Therapies—Consensus Recommendations. Plast Reconstr Surg 2008;121(5):5S–30S.
6. Niamtu J III. Filler injection with micro-cannula instead of needles. Dermatol Surg 2009;35(12): 2005–8.
7. Tatjana Pavicic KF, Erlbacher K, Neuner R, et al. Precision in Dermal Filling: A Comparison Between Needle and Cannula When Using Soft Tissue Fillers. J Drugs Dermatol JDD 2017;16(9):866–72.
8. van Loghem JA, Humzah D, Kerscher M. Cannula versus sharp needle for placement of soft tissue fillers: an observational cadaver study. Aesthetic Surg J 2018;38(1):73–88.
9. Jewell ML. Commentary on: Cannula vs Sharp Needle for Placement of Soft Tissue Fillers: An Observational Cadaver Study. Aesthet Surg J 2017;38(1): 89–91.
10. Griepentrog GJ, Lemke BN, Burkat CN, et al. Anatomical position of hyaluronic Acid gel following injection to the infraorbital hollows. Ophthalmic Plast Reconstr Surg 2013;29(1):35–9.
11. Ahramiyanpour N, Rastaghi F, Parvar SY, et al. Subcision in acne scarring: a review of clinical trials. J Cosmet Dermatol 2023;22(3):744–51.
12. Ebrahim HM, Nassar A, ElKashishy K, et al. A combined approach of subcision with either cross-linked hyaluronic acid or threads in the treatment of atrophic acne scars. J Cosmet Dermatol 2022;21(8):3334–42.
13. Casabona G. Blood aspiration test for cosmetic fillers to prevent accidental intravascular injection in the face. Dermatol Surg 2015;41(7):841–7.
14. Goodman GJ, Magnusson MR, Callan P, et al. A consensus on minimizing the risk of hyaluronic acid embolic visual loss and suggestions for immediate bedside management. Aesthetic Surg J 2020; 40(9):1009–21.
15. Fulton J, Caperton C, Weinkle S, et al. Filler injections with the blunt-tip microcannula. J Drugs Dermatol JDD: J Drugs Dermatol JDD 2012;11(9):1098–103.
16. Kisyova R, Karkhi A, Lalemi C. Using a needle versus cannula: the advantages and disadvantages. Journal of Aesthetic Nursing 2020;9(2):81–3.
17. Tansatit T, Apinuntrum P, Phetudom T. A dark side of the cannula injections: how arterial wall perforations and emboli occur. Aesthetic Plast Surg 2017;41:221–7.
18. Ugradar S, Hoenig J. Measurement of the force required by blunt-tipped microcannulas to perforate the facial artery. Ophthalmic Plast Reconstr Surg 2019;35(5):444–6.
19. Raspaldo H. Volumizing effect of a new hyaluronic acid sub-dermal facial filler: a retrospective analysis based on 102 cases. J Cosmet Laser Ther 2008; 10(3):134–42.
20. Funt D, Pavicic T. Dermal fillers in aesthetics: an overview of adverse events and treatment approaches. Clin Cosmet Invest Dermatol 2013;6:295–316.
21. DeLorenzi C. Complications of injectable fillers, part I. Aesthetic Surg J 2013;33(4):561–75.
22. Kuldeep Singh SN. Nonvascular Complications of Injectable Fillers— Prevention and Management. Indian J Plast Surg 2020;53:335–43.

23. Murad Alam RK, Dover Jeffrey S, Harikumar Vishnu, et al. Rates of Vascular Occlusion Associated With Using Needles vs Cannulas for Filler Injection. JAMA Dermatology 2021;157:174–80.
24. Beleznay K, Carruthers JD, Humphrey S, et al. Avoiding and treating blindness from fillers: a review of the world literature. Dermatol Surg 2015;41(10):1097–117.
25. DeLorenzi C. Complications of injectable fillers, part 2: vascular complications. Aesthetic Surg J 2014;34(4):584–600.
26. Pavicic T, Webb KL, Frank K, et al. Arterial wall penetration forces in needles versus cannulas. Plast Reconstr Surg 2019;143(3):504e–12e.
27. Coleman SR. Avoidance of arterial occlusion from injection of soft tissue fillers. Aesthetic Surg J 2002;22(6):555–7.
28. Khan TT, Colon-Acevedo B, Mettu P, et al. An anatomical analysis of the supratrochlear artery: considerations in facial filler injections and preventing vision loss. Aesthetic Surg J 2017;37(2):203–8.
29. Cohen JL, Biesman BS, Dayan SH, et al. Treatment of hyaluronic acid filler–induced impending necrosis with hyaluronidase: consensus recommendations. Aesthetic Surg J 2015;35(7):844–9.
30. van Loghem J, Sattler S, Casabona G, et al. Consensus on the use of hyaluronic acid fillers from the cohesive polydensified matrix range: best practice in specific facial indications. Clin Cosmet Invest Dermatol 2021;1175–99.
31. Juhász MLW, Marmur ES. Temporal fossa defects: techniques for injecting hyaluronic acid filler and complications after hyaluronic acid filler injection. J Cosmet Dermatol 2015;14(3):254–9.
32. Beer JI, Sieber DA, Scheuer JF III, et al. Three-dimensional facial anatomy: structure and function as it relates to injectable neuromodulators and soft tissue fillers. Plastic and Reconstructive Surgery Global Open 2016;4(12 Suppl). https://doi.org/10.1097/GOX.0000000000001175.
33. Bass LS. Injectable filler techniques for facial rejuvenation, volumization, and augmentation. Facial Plast Surg Clin 2015;23(4):479–88.
34. Hexsel D, Soirefmann M, Donida Porto M, et al. Double-Blind, Randomized, Controlled Clinical Trial to Compare Safety and Efficacy of a Metallic Cannula with that of a Standard Needle for Soft Tissue Augmentation of the Nasolabial Folds. Dermatol Surg 2012;38(2 Part 1):207–14.
35. Walker L, Cetto R. Lip Augmentation Using Hyaluronic Acid Filler and a 4-mm Needle: A Safer, More Natural, and Predictable Approach. J Clin Aesthet Dermatol 2021;14(1). E61–e63.
36. Surek CC, Guisantes E, Schnarr K, et al. "No-touch" technique for lip enhancement. Plast Reconstr Surg 2016;138(4):603e–13e.

Clinical Assessment, Diagnosis, and Management of Infraorbital Wrinkles and Pigmentation

Gyanesh Rathore, MD[a], Kinnor Das, MD[b], Marina Landau, MD[c],
Ines Verner, MD[d], Martin Kassir, MD[e], Hassan I. Galadari, MD[f],
Michael H. Gold, MD[g], Mahsa Babaei, MD[h], Mohamad Goldust, MD[i],*

KEYWORDS

- Infraorbital wrinkle • Infraorbital pigmentation • Peeling • Microneedling • Laser therapy
- Cosmetic dermatology

KEY POINTS

- Infraorbital wrinkle and pigmentation is a common cosmetic concern.
- Factors, including genetics, aging, sun exposure, lack of sleep, stress, and hormonal changes, can cause infraorbital wrinkle and pigmentation.
- The diagnosis is usually based on a clinical examination.
- Treatment depends on the underlying cause and severity of the condition. Topical lightening agents, chemical peels, laser therapy, microneedling, and lifestyle changes as well as more-invasive methods, including surgeries, are among the prescribed options.

INTRODUCTION

The skin around the eyes is one of the most highly sensitive areas of the face that is susceptible to senility and senescence, resulting in wrinkles and hyperpigmentation. This is mainly due to the specific structure of the skin and subcutaneous tissue in this area. Infraorbital wrinkles are induced by repetitive skin contracture, sun and pollutant exposure, smoking, and hormonal status. Infraorbital pigmentation is a common cosmetic and dermatologic concern, characterized by the appearance of darkening of the skin as well as brownish discoloration of the skin. Numerous variables, including ancestry, age, sun exposure, sleep deprivation, and stress, contribute to this condition. The dark area of the skin below the eyes can make a person look tired and older, and subsequently, decrease their self-esteem. With the increasing interest in skincare and antiaging, many individuals are seeking treatments for infraorbital wrinkle and pigmentation.[1–3]

This review examines the underlying pathophysiology, related causes, associated symptoms and concerns, prevention, and management of infraorbital wrinkle and pigmentation, using the currently available knowledge, including clinical studies and available products.

EPIDEMIOLOGY

Pigmentation under the eyes is a common cosmetic issue that affects individuals of all ages and all

[a] Department of Dermatology, Military Hospital, Dimapur, Nagaland, India; [b] Apollo Clinic, Silchar, Assam, India; [c] Department of Plastic Surgery, Shamir Medical Center, Be'er Ya'akov, Israel; [d] Verner Clinic for Dermatology and Aesthetics, Tel Aviv, Israel; [e] Worldwide Laser Institute, Dallas, USA; [f] College of Medicine and Health Sciences, United Arab Emirates University, Al Ain, United Arab Emirates; [g] Gold Skin Care Center, Tennessee Clinical Research Center, Nashville, TN, USA; [h] School of Medicine, Stanford University, Stanford, CA, USA; [i] Department of Dermatology, Yale University School of Medicine, New Haven, CT 06510, USA
* Corresponding author.
E-mail address: mohamad.goldust@yale.edu

Dermatol Clin 42 (2024) 79–88
https://doi.org/10.1016/j.det.2023.07.005
0733-8635/24/© 2023 Elsevier Inc. All rights reserved.

skin types. Because melanin-rich skin is more prone to hyperpigmentation, it is more common in those with darker skin tones. The incidence of infraorbital pigmentation increases with age, and it is estimated to affect up to 50% of people aged 50 years and above.[1] Interestingly, studies have also reported that the incidence of infraorbital pigmentation gradually increases without any intervention. Therefore, early intervention and management are highly recommended.[4–6] In addition to pigmentation, those who are older are more likely to have infraorbital wrinkles.[2] According to the literature, higher rates of infraorbital wrinkles among older adults are attributed to higher rates of bone resorption, fat atrophy, and laxity of muscles and ligaments among them.[3] Moreover, although infraorbital wrinkles are more prevalent among women than among men, it depends on several clinical, behavioral, and psychological elements, including body mass index, alcohol use, smoking, and socioeconomic strata. Studies have also reported that the incidence of infraorbital pigmentation gradually increases without any intervention. Therefore, early intervention and management are highly recommended.[4–6]

CAUSE

Infraorbital wrinkling is part of the normal aging process, but can worsen. Infraorbital wrinkles and pigmentation can be caused by several different factors. The skin around the eyes is fragile and thin and is poor in sebaceous glands, making it highly vulnerable to the effects of aging and environmental factors. Several prevalent dermatoses are commonly associated with infraorbital wrinkling and pigmentation. Periorbital darkness can be due to melanosis (gray-brown color), vascular (blue/pink/purple color), or structural. The structural type can be associated with infraorbital palpebral bags, blepharoptosis, and loss of fat with bony prominence.

Atopic Dermatitis

This skin condition can cause itching, redness, and swelling around the eyes, leading to wrinkles and pigmentation. The latter is due to a postinflammatory reaction.[7]

Contact Dermatitis

Contact with irritants, such as cosmetic products, sunscreens, and other skincare products, can cause inflammation, dark circles, and wrinkles around the eyes.[7]

Psoriasis

This autoimmune skin condition can cause patches of red, scaly skin that can be itchy and painful, making the skin around the eyes highly susceptible to developing wrinkles and pigmentation.[7]

Melasma

This skin condition is caused by overproduction of melanin and can result in dark pigmentation around the eyes.[7]

Periorbital Hyperpigmentation

The skin around the eyes darkens, leaving wrinkles and dark circles behind. According to Sawant and Khan,[8] there are intrinsic (internal) and extrinsic (external) reasons for periorbital hyperpigmentation. Intrinsic factors include genetics, aging, hormonal changes, and medical conditions, such as allergies, sinusitis, and eczema, whereas extrinsic factors include sun exposure, environmental pollution, stress, and lack of sleep.[4,5]

Aging

As people get older, the skin loses its suppleness and collagen content, which leads to the onset of wrinkles and sagging. In addition, changes in hormone levels, such as estrogenic depletion during menopause, can also contribute to the formation of wrinkles.[9]

Sun Exposure

UV rays from the sun can also cause damage to the skin, leading to the development of wrinkles and pigmentation. Sun exposure triggers the production of melanin. UV radiation stimulates melanocytes to produce more melanin, resulting in the appearance of dark circles under the eyes. This pigmentation is most commonly seen in people with darker skin, whereas people with lighter skin are more susceptible to sun damage and wrinkles. In addition to pigmentation, UV radiation breaks down collagen and elastin, 2 proteins that contribute to elasticity and firmness of the skin leading to wrinkles, fine lines, and sagging skin.[10–12]

Studies have found that exposure to UV radiation is an important cause of skin aging, which can lead to the development of premature aging signs and wrinkles under the eyes.[13] It was found that UV exposure from sun rays is a key factor in the development of under-eye wrinkles, and that wearing sunglasses and applying a broad-spectrum sunscreen can help protect the sensitive skin around the eyes from sun damage. This area is also exposed to sun more than many other parts of the body owing to the anatomy and location, increasing the risk of sun exposure within this area.[9]

Lifestyle Habits

Lifestyle habits, such as smoking, alcohol consumption, and poor diet, can also contribute to the formation of wrinkles and pigmentation specifically in the skin surrounding the eyes. Multiple studies have found that smoking, in particular, has been shown to cause the skin to age faster, leading to the development of wrinkles.[14–17]

Genetics

Wrinkles and pigmentation around the eyes may also be influenced by genetics. Certain people are more prone to developing wrinkles and pigmentation compared with others.[18]

CLINICAL AND LABORATORY ASSESSMENT

The diagnosis of infraorbital pigmentation is usually based on a clinical examination, and there are no specific tests required to confirm the diagnosis. However, some tests can help confirm the cause of the condition.

Wood Lamp

This diagnostic tool is used in dermatology to examine the skin and hair for various conditions. In the case of infraorbital pigmentation, it can be used to differentiate between various types of hyperpigmentation of different origins, such as melasma, postinflammatory hyperpigmentation (PIH), and aging-related spots. When examining the infraorbital area with a Wood lamp, the light illuminates the skin and causes the pigmented cells to fluoresce, allowing the dermatologist to see the distribution and depth of the pigmentation. Melasma, for example, appears as a light brown or gray fluorescence, while age spots appear as yellow fluorescence. PIH appears as a more diffuse fluorescence without any clear pattern. By using a Wood lamp, dermatologists can determine the type of pigmentation and develop a treatment plan accordingly. This tool is also helpful in monitoring clinical progress following treatment. It is important to note that a Wood lamp examination is only one part of a comprehensive evaluation of infraorbital pigmentation and should be used in conjunction with other diagnostic tools and techniques.[19–21]

Biopsy

In some cases, a physician may perform a skin biopsy to rule out other underlying medical conditions, such as atopic or contact dermatitis. This can aid in the development of an effective treatment plan.[22–24]

Dermoscopy

Dermoscopy is a noninvasive diagnostic method used to examine the skin in detail, including pigmented lesions. This method can be especially useful in the diagnosis of infraorbital pigmentation. A dermatoscope magnifies the skin and allows the physician to see the structure and texture of the skin in more detail. The dermatoscope emits polarized light, which helps in detecting any abnormalities that may be contributing to pigmentation. Multiple recent studies have shown that dermatoscopy is a valuable tool, allowing an accurate diagnosis and appropriate treatment of the condition.[25–28]

TYPES OF THE DISORDER

Recently, Huang and colleagues[29] performed a clinical analysis and proposed classification of infraorbital pigmentation on the basis of clinical presentation. Periorbital hyperpigmentation was classified into pigmented, vascular, structural, and mixed type.

Wrinkles under the eyes can be classified as static or dynamic.[30,31] Dynamic wrinkles are formed owing to repetitive skin contracture following periorbital muscle activity.[31,32] Static wrinkles are due to chronologic aging of the skin or to aging induced by exogenous factors, such as sun exposure or smoking. They demonstrate specific histologic alterations. In addition, under the eyes, because of specific anatomic characteristics, "pseudowrinkles" can be seen. Those are formed because of decreased function of the epidermal barrier, causing water loss from the epidermis. These wrinkles disappear with adequate skin hydration.[33]

PREVENTION

Preventing infraorbital wrinkles and pigmentation is important in maintaining a youthful and healthy appearance. Several methods that can help prevent the development of infraorbital wrinkles and pigmentation are listed in later discussion.

Sun Protection

Wearing sun protection on a daily basis, in the form of sunglasses in addition to a broad-spectrum sunscreen, can help to prevent the damaging effects of UV rays on the skin.[34]

Diet

A study has shown that a diet rich in antioxidants and anti-inflammatory foods, such as fruits and vegetables, can decrease the chance for the development of infraorbital wrinkles and pigmentation.[35]

Avoid Smoking and Excessive Alcohol Consumption

Smoking and excessive alcohol consumption can cause damage to the skin, leading to the development of wrinkles and pigmentation.[15,17]

Getting Adequate Sleep

Getting adequate sleep can help to reduce the appearance of wrinkles and dark circles around the eyes.[36]

Active Medical and Cosmetic Ingredients

Adequate skin hydration is of uppermost importance to prevent infraorbital pseudowrinkles. In addition, topical agents containing tretinoin are also important.[37,38]

TREATMENT

The underlying cause and degree of infraorbital pigmentation determine the appropriate course of therapy. Some of the management options include the following.

Topical Treatments

These agents contain active ingredients, such as hydroquinone, kojic acid, or azelaic acid, that help with reduction of melanin production, and therefore, brighten the skin.[39]

Retinoids

The antiaging benefits of topical retinoids like retinol and tretinoin are well established. They boost collagen synthesis, reduce wrinkles and fine lines, and level out skin tone.[40] Care should be taken when using these agents, as irritation to skin is common, which can further worsen the condition.

Vitamin C

As a potent antioxidant, vitamin C helps prevent free radical damage to the skin and encourages skin cell renewal. The look of fine lines and wrinkles may be improved, and dark infraorbital circles can be brightened with topical vitamin C. Derivatives of ascorbic acid, including L-ascorbic acid 6-palmitate and magnesium ascorbyl phosphate, are used in cosmetic formulations because of ascorbic acid's instability in many topical applications. The main antioxidant in the skin is L-ascorbic acid. Free radicals that might cause the development of melanin in the aqueous compartment are neutralized by it. In addition, vitamin C increases the formation of collagen and masks the hue of stagnant blood, which might make dark circles beneath the eyes look better.

In a split-face study done in 2009 by Ohshima and colleagues,[41] they concluded that melanin production in human melanocytes can be suppressed by vitamin C as well as by its derivatives, such as magnesium ascorbyl phosphate and ascorbic acid glucoside. Two different types of 10% vitamin C lotions were used on opposite sides of the face to treat dark circles. One side was treated with sodium ascorbate, while the other was treated with ascorbic acid glucoside. The researchers measured the melanin index, erythema index, thickness, and echogenicity of the skin on both eyelids and found that the pigmentation was reduced as a result of the increased skin thickness, leading to hiding of the dark discoloration from congested blood. However, they did not observe a significant change in the melanin index.

Niacinamide

Niacinamide is a form of vitamin B3 that has been shown to improve skin hydration and elasticity. It can also help to lighten hyperpigmentation by suppressing the transfer of melanosomes to keratinocytes and improve the overall appearance of the under-eye area.[42]

Peptides

Small chains of amino acids called peptides have been shown to increase skin firmness and collagen synthesis. Infraorbital wrinkles and fine lines are subject to look less noticeable using topical peptides. Because of their potential to impact melanogenesis, they can contribute to skin lightening.[43,44]

Kojic Acid

Kojic acid is a natural ingredient that has been shown to lighten hyperpigmentation and even out skin tone.[45] In addition, it might aid in minimizing the appearance of fine lines and wrinkles around the eyes.[46]

Arbutin

Arbutin is a type of herbal extract obtained from the leaves of plants, such as bearberry, cranberry, pear, and blueberry. It has the ability to inhibit tyrosine activity and therefore prevents melanosome maturation, but its effects are dependent on the dose.[47] Higher concentrations may result in hyperpigmentation, which needs further investigation.[48] It is commercially available in a 3% concentration. A gel containing topical arbutin was found to be effective in reducing pigmentation in individuals with melasma in a randomized open study conducted by Ertam and colleagues.[49]

Hyaluronic Acid

Hyaluronic acid is a naturally occurring substance that helps to hydrate the skin and improve its plumpness. Topical hyaluronic acid or in the form of microneedle patches can help to reduce the appearance of infraorbital wrinkles and fine lines.[50,51]

Azelaic Acid

Azelaic acid, also known as 1,7-heptanedicarboxylic acid, was originally created as a topical medication for acne treatment. However, because of its ability to impact tyrosine, it has also been used in the management of hyperpigmentation conditions like melasma.[52–54] The way it works is by inhibiting DNA synthesis and mitochondrial enzymes, leading to direct harm to the melanocyte cells. It has been shown in vitro to disrupt DNA synthesis and mitochondrial enzymes in abnormal melanocytes and fibroblasts, making it safe for long-term use without the risk of leukoderma or exogenous ochronosis.[53] Its effectiveness in treating facial PIH makes it a promising candidate for treating periocular pigmentation.[54,55]

Chemical Peels

Exfoliation brought on by chemical peels aids in removing the top layer of skin and reveals a more radiant complexion. Chemical peels may be used to treat pigmentation and infraorbital wrinkles, 2 prevalent cosmetic issues. This encourages cell regeneration and reveals a smoother, more luminous complexion. Chemical peels come in a variety of forms, each with a unique active component and intensity. The following describes the function of several chemical peels in the treatment of infraorbital wrinkles and discoloration.

Alpha-hydroxy acid (AHA) peels

AHAs are a group of naturally occurring acids that are commonly used in skincare products, including peels. They are known for their exfoliating and skin-renewing properties, which can help improve the appearance of fine lines, wrinkles, and hyperpigmentation, including the infraorbital area. AHAs, such as glycolic acid and lactic acid, are mild exfoliating agents that penetrate the uppermost layer of skin, helping to reduce fine lines and wrinkles, improve texture, and brighten pigmentation. AHA peels are often recommended for those with sensitive skin or as a starting point for those new to chemical peels.

Studies have shown that AHAs can help to increase collagen production, which gives skin its firmness and elasticity, and can also help to improve the overall texture and tone of the skin.[56] AHAs can also help to lighten dark infraorbital circles by breaking down melanin.[57] It is important to note that AHA peels should be used with caution, as they can cause skin irritation and sensitivity in some individuals, especially those with sensitive skin.[58] Before using an AHA peel, it is recommended to patch test on a small area of skin to check for any adverse reactions.[59,60]

Beta-hydroxy acid (BHA) or salicylic acid peels

BHA peels are a type of chemical peel used for exfoliating the skin and improving the appearance of infraorbital wrinkles and pigmentation. BHAs are oil-soluble, making them ideal for use on oily skin or in areas where sebum buildup is more common, such as under the eyes. BHAs, such as salicylic acid, are oil-soluble and can penetrate deeper into the pores to help unclog them and reduce acne.[61] BHAs can also help to lighten infraorbital pigmentation and improve the overall texture and tone of the skin.[62–67]

Jessner peels

Jessner peels are a combination of salicylic acid (14%), lactic acid (14%), and resorcinol (14%) usually in equal concentrations. They are more potent than AHAs and can provide more significant improvement in fine lines, wrinkles, and hyperpigmentation, especially for those with more resilient skin. Studies have shown that the Jessner peel can be effective in reducing the appearance of infraorbital wrinkles and pigmentation.[68,69]

Trichloroacetic acid (TCA) peels

TCA peels can be used as superficial or medium-depth peels depending on TCA concentration in the solution. At higher TCA concentrations, TCA can penetrate through the outer layer of the skin and into the reticular dermis for a medium-depth peel. They are effective in reducing deeper wrinkles, hyperpigmentation, and acne scars.[68,70] TCA peels are more potent and require more recovery time than AHAs or BHAs and should be performed by an experienced professional. TCA is applied to the skin in a thin layer and works by causing a controlled injury to the skin. This leads to the stimulation of new skin growth and the formation of collagen, which is an important protein for skin elasticity.[71] TCA peels also remove the top layer of skin, which can help to smooth out fine lines and wrinkles around the eyes. It is also effective in treating infraorbital pigmentation because it can remove hyperpigmented skin cells that contribute to discoloration. The peel can also stimulate the production of new skin cells, which can help to even out skin tone.[72] It is important to note that TCA peels can cause side effects, such as redness, swelling, and peeling, so it is important to counsel patients about these side effects in detail, before the procedure. In addition, individuals with sensitive skin or any concurrent inflammatory skin conditions, such as rosacea or eczema, may not be suitable candidates for TCA peels.[73]

Phenol peels

Phenol peels are the strongest and most potent type of chemical peel. They are typically used for severe cases of skin aging, sun damage, and hyperpigmentation and penetrate the deepest layers of skin. Phenol peels are generally performed under sedation and can cause significant redness and discomfort during the healing process.[74–76]

Laser Therapy

Laser therapy uses high-intensity light to target the pigment in the skin, breaking it down and eventually fading the dark circles. Lasers have become an increasingly popular method for treating infraorbital wrinkles and pigmentation. Different types of lasers are used for various skin concerns, including fine lines, dark circles, and hyperpigmentation.

Fractional CO_2 lasers

This type of laser is commonly used for the treatment of fine lines and wrinkles under the eyes. The laser creates tiny, microscopic wounds on the skin, which trigger the body's natural healing process, resulting in new, healthy skin growth. The fractional CO_2 laser is particularly effective for treating deep wrinkles and fine lines.[77]

Nd:YAG laser

This type of laser is often used for the treatment of hyperpigmentation and dark circles under the eyes. The Nd:YAG laser emits energy into the skin, which is absorbed by the melanin and breaks it down, resulting in a reduction of dark circles and hyperpigmentation.[78]

Erbium lasers

This type of laser is also used for treating fine lines and wrinkles under the eyes. The Erbium laser is similar to the fractional CO_2 laser, but it uses a different wavelength of light that is less invasive, making it a good option for those with sensitive skin.[79]

Intense pulsed light (IPL)

IPL is commonly used for treating dark circles and hyperpigmentation under the eyes. The IPL laser uses high-intensity pulses of light to penetrate the skin and target the melanin, resulting in a reduction of dark circles and hyperpigmentation.[80,81]

Microneedling

Microneedling is a minimally invasive procedure that stimulates collagen production and improves the skin's texture and tone. Microneedling is a cosmetic procedure that involves using fine needles to create tiny punctures in the skin, triggering the skin's natural healing process. This procedure has been found to be effective in managing infraorbital wrinkles and pigmentation. The role of microneedling in the management of infraorbital wrinkles and pigmentation is to stimulate the skin's natural healing process and increase the production of collagen and elastin, the 2 key proteins responsible for maintaining skin elasticity and firmness.[81] This can help to reduce the appearance of wrinkles and improve skin texture and tone, reducing the visibility of pigmentation. In addition, microneedling can also improve the penetration and effectiveness of topical skincare products, further enhancing the results of the treatment.[82,83] There are several methods of microneedling that can be used to target infraorbital wrinkles and pigmentation. Microneedling is not a one-time solution, and several visits are needed to gain favorable clinical outcome. It is also important to explain the posttreatment care to the patient to ensure safe and effective treatment. Microneedling can be performed manually or by using energy-based devices, such as radiofrequency, which is commonly being used.[84]

Other Interventional Methods Include the Following

Blepharoplasty and brow lift

These procedures remove excessive skin, fat, and muscle from the upper or lower eyelids to improve the appearance of wrinkles. This procedure involves lifting the eyebrows to reduce the appearance of wrinkles in the forehead and under the eyes.[85,86]

Botulinum toxin injections

This procedure involves injecting a small amount of botulinum toxin into the muscles that cause wrinkles to reduce the movement of these muscles and smooth out the wrinkles. However, the results are not permanent, and regular sessions are necessary in order to maintain the desired results.[87,88]

Fat transfer

This procedure involves transferring fat from another part of the body to the infraorbital area to fill in wrinkles and hollows.[89]

Soft tissue filler injections

Soft tissue filler injections: This procedure involves injecting fillers into the infraorbital area to add volume and smooth out wrinkles. It also helps fade the infraorbital pigmentation. Most commonly used preparations involve hyaluronic acid fillers.[90,91]

Lifestyle changes

Lifestyle changes play a crucial role in the prevention of infraorbital wrinkles and pigmentation.[14] Some of the key lifestyle changes that can help prevent these skin concerns include the following.

Sleep
Adequate sleep is essential for skin health, as it helps repair and rejuvenate the skin. Lack of sleep can lead to dark circles, infraorbital wrinkles, and pigmentation.

Hydration
Staying hydrated is crucial for healthy skin. Infraorbital skin should be constantly hydrated by using appropriate topical moisturizing products, especially in aged individuals, in whom epidermal skin barrier usually malfunctions.

Sun protection
Exposure to UV rays from the sun can cause skin damage, leading to wrinkles and pigmentation. Wearing sunscreen and protective clothing can help prevent these skin concerns. Multiple studies published have found that daily sun protection significantly reduced the appearance of wrinkles and pigmentation.

Healthy diet
Eating a diet rich in vitamins, minerals, and antioxidants can help prevent skin damage and promote skin health. Studies have found that a diet rich in antioxidants and anti-inflammatory foods can help prevent skin aging and pigmentation.

Stress management
Stress can lead to skin aging and pigmentation. Practicing stress-management techniques, like meditation and yoga, can help reduce stress levels, promoting skin health.

SUMMARY

Infraorbital wrinkle and pigmentation is a common cosmetic concern that can be induced by many different factors, such as genetics, aging, sun exposure, lack of sleep, stress, and hormonal changes. The diagnosis is usually based on a clinical examination, and the treatment depends on the underlying cause and severity of the condition. Topical lightening agents, chemical peels, laser therapy, microneedling, and lifestyle changes as well as more-invasive methods, including surgeries, are some of the most commonly prescribed treatments for the management of infraorbital wrinkle and pigmentation.

CLINICS CARE POINTS

- Factors, including genetics, aging, sun exposure, lack of sleep, stress, and hormonal changes, can cause infraorbital wrinkle and pigmentation.
- Investigation of the exact underlying pathophysiology and development of more targeted therapies are highly recommended to future researchers.
- More accurate studies are needd to develop meticulous diagnostic and therapeutic guidlines, based on patient's age, gender and race for the treatment of this disorder.

DISCLOSURE

None of the authors have any conflict of interest for this submission.

SOURCES OF SUPPORT IF ANY

None.

DISCLAIMER

The authors confirm that the article has been read and approved by all the authors, that the requirements for authorship as stated earlier in this document have been met and that each author believes that the article represents honest work.

REFERENCES

1. Nouveau S, Agrawal D, Kohli M, et al. Skin Hyperpigmentation in Indian Population: Insights and Best Practice. Indian J Dermatol 2016;61(5):487–95.
2. Manríquez JJ, Cataldo K, Vera-Kellet C, et al. Wrinkles. Clin Evid 2014;2014:1711.
3. Arora G, Arora S. Periorbital rejuvenation: A study on the use of dermal threads as monotherapy, with a review of literature. J Cutan Aesthetic Surg 2022; 15:48.
4. Ranu H, Thng S, Goh BK, et al. Periorbital Hyperpigmentation in Asians: An Epidemiologic Study and a Proposed Classification. Dermatol Surg 2011;37: 1297–303.
5. David BG, Roshini RM, Shankar R. A clinico-epidemiological study of periorbital melanosis. Int J Res Dermatol 2017;3:245.
6. Roberts WE. Periorbital hyperpigmentation: review of etiology, medical evaluation, and aesthetic treatment. J Drugs Dermatol JDD 2014;13:472–82.

7. Freitag FM, Cestari TF. What causes dark circles under the eyes. J Cosmet Dermatol 2007;6:211–5.

8. Sawant O, Khan T. Management of periorbital hyperpigmentation: An overview of nature-based agents and alternative approaches. Dermatol Ther 2020;33.

9. Sanches Silveira JEP, Myaki Pedroso DM. UV light and skin aging. Rev Environ Health 2014;29.

10. Roh MR, Chung KY. Infraorbital Dark Circles: Definition, Causes, and Treatment Options. Dermatol Surg 2009;35:1163–71.

11. Imokawa G, Ishida K. Biological Mechanisms Underlying the Ultraviolet Radiation-Induced Formation of Skin Wrinkling and Sagging I: Reduced Skin Elasticity, Highly Associated with Enhanced Dermal Elastase Activity, Triggers Wrinkling and Sagging. Indian J Manag Sci 2015;16:7753–75.

12. Akiba S, Shinkura R, Miyamoto K, et al. Influence of Chronic UV Exposure and Lifestyle on Facial Skin Photo-Aging –Results from a Pilot Study. J Epidemiol 1999;9:136–42.

13. Rabe JH, Mamelak AJ, McElgunn PJS, et al. Photoaging: Mechanisms and repair. J Am Acad Dermatol 2006;55:1–19.

14. Hamer MA, Pardo LM, Jacobs LC, et al. Lifestyle and Physiological Factors Associated with Facial Wrinkling in Men and Women. J Invest Dermatol 2017;137(8):1692–9.

15. Koh JS, Kang H, Choi SW, et al. Cigarette smoking associated with premature facial wrinkling: image analysis of facial skin replicas. Int J Dermatol 2002;41:21–7.

16. Schnohr P, Lange P, Nyboe J, et al. [Does smoking increase the degree of wrinkles on the face. The Osterbro study]. Ugeskr Laeger 1991;153:660–2.

17. Kadunce DP. Cigarette Smoking: Risk Factor for Premature Facial Wrinkling. Ann Intern Med 1991;114:840.

18. Chen Y, André M, Adhikari K, et al. A genome-wide association study identifies novel gene associations with facial skin wrinkling and mole count in Latin Americans. Br J Dermatol 2021;185(5):988–98.

19. Asawanonda P, Taylor CR. Wood's light in dermatology. Int J Dermatol 1999;38:801–7.

20. Gilchrest BA, Fitzpatrick TB, Anderson RR, et al. Localization of melanin pigmentation in the skin with Wood's lamp. Br J Dermatol 1977;96:245–8.

21. Sarkar R, Das A. Periorbital Hyperpigmentation: What Lies Beneath? Indian Dermatol Online J 2018;9:229–30.

22. Goodman RM. Periorbital Hyperpigmentation: An Overlooked Genetic Disorder of Pigmentation. Arch Dermatol 1969;100:169.

23. Nayak CS, Giri AS, Zambare US. A Study of Clinico-pathological Correlation of Periorbital Hyperpigmentation. Indian Dermatol Online J 2018;9:245–9.

24. Ing EB, Buncic JR, Weiser BA, et al. Periorbital hyperpigmentation and erythema dyschromicum perstans. Can J Ophthalmol 1992;27:353–5.

25. Mahesh AR, Arumilli KPP, Kotha S, et al. Clinical and Dermoscopic Evaluation of Periorbital Melanosis. J Cutan Aesthet Surg 2022;15(2):154–60.

26. Ramakrishnan S, Hegde SP, Shenoy MM, et al. A cross-sectional study on clinico-dermoscopic features of periorbital melanosis in a tertiary care hospital. J Cosmet Dermatol 2021;20(9):2917–23.

27. Chhabra N, Khare S, Sachdev D. Dermoscopy as an efficient aid to diagnose pigmentary and vascular component of periorbital melanosis: A cross-sectional study. J Cosmet Dermatol 2022;21:5880–6.

28. Ahuja S, Deshmukh A, Khushalani S. A study of dermatoscopic pattern of periorbital hypermelanosis. Pigment Int 2017;4:29.

29. Huang YL, Chang SL, Ma L, et al. Clinical analysis and classification of dark eye circle. Int J Dermatol 2014;53(2):164–70.

30. Kligman AM, Zheng P, Lavker RM. The anatomy and pathogenesis of wrinkles. Br J Dermatol 1985;113:37–42.

31. Fujimura T, Hotta M. The preliminary study of the relationship between facial movements and wrinkle formation. Skin Res Technol 2012;18:219–24.

32. Stutman RL, Codner MA. Tear Trough Deformity: Review of Anatomy and Treatment Options. Aesthetic Surg J 2012;32:426–40.

33. Tsuji T, Yorifuji T, Hayashi Y, et al. Light and scanning electron microscopic studies on wrinkles in aged persons' skin. Br J Dermatol 1986 Mar;114(3):329–35.

34. Behar-Cohen F, Baillet G, de Ayguavives T, et al. Ultraviolet damage to the eye revisited: eye-sun protection factor (E-SPF®), a new ultraviolet protection label for eyewear. Clin Ophthlmol 2013. https://doi.org/10.2147/OPTH.S46189.

35. Geng R, Kang S-G, Huang K, et al. Boosting the Photoaged Skin: The Potential Role of Dietary Components. Nutrients 2021;13:1691.

36. Sundelin T, Lekander M, Kecklund G, et al. Cues of fatigue: effects of sleep deprivation on facial appearance. Sleep 2013;36(9):1355–60.

37. Nguyen TQ, Zahr AS, Kononov T, et al. A Randomized, Double-blind, Placebo-controlled Clinical Study Investigating the Efficacy and Tolerability of a Peptide Serum Targeting Expression Lines. J Clin Aesthet Dermatol 2021;14:14–21.

38. Jagdeo J, Kurtti A, Hernandez S, et al. Novel Vitamin C and E and Green Tea Polyphenols Combination Serum Improves Photoaged Facial Skin. J Drugs Dermatol JDD 2021;20:996–1003.

39. Rendon MI, Gaviria JI. Review of Skin-Lightning Agents. Dermatol Surg 2006;31:886–90.

40. Ortonne J-P. Retinoid therapy of pigmentary disorders. Dermatol Ther 2006;19:280–8.

41. Ohshima H, Mizukoshi K, Oyobikawa M, et al. Effects of vitamin C on dark circles of the lower eyelids: quantitative evaluation using image analysis and echogram. Skin Res Technol 2009;15(2):214–7.

42. Hakozaki T, Minwalla L, Zhuang J, et al. The effect of niacinamide on reducing cutaneous pigmentation and suppression of melanosome transfer. Br J Dermatol 2002;147:20–31.

43. Farwick M, Maczkiewitz U, Lersch P, et al. Facial skin-lightning benefits of the tetrapeptide Pro-Lys-Glu-Lys on subjects with skin types V-VI living in South Africa: Skin-lightning benefits of PKEK. J Cosmet Dermatol 2011;10:217–23.

44. Gillbro JM, Olsson MJ. The melanogenesis and mechanisms of skin-lightning agents - existing and new approaches: Melanogenesis and skin-lightning agents. Int J Cosmet Sci 2011;33:210–21.

45. Phasha V, Senabe J, Ndzotoyi P, et al. Review on the Use of Kojic Acid—A Skin-Lightning Ingredient. Cosmetics 2022;9(3):64.

46. Gonçalez ML, Corrêa MA, Chorilli M. Skin Delivery of Kojic Acid-Loaded Nanotechnology-Based Drug Delivery Systems for the Treatment of Skin Aging. BioMed Res Int 2013;1–9.

47. Boo YC. Arbutin as a Skin Depigmenting Agent with Antimelanogenic and Antioxidant Properties. Antioxidants 2021;10:1129.

48. Davis EC, Callender VD. Postinflammatory hyperpigmentation: a review of the epidemiology, clinical features, and treatment options in skin of color. J Clin Aesthet Dermatol 2010;3:20–31.

49. Ertam I, Mutlu B, Unal I, et al. Efficiency of ellagic acid and arbutin in melasma: a randomized, prospective, open-label study. J Dermatol 2008;35(9): 570–4.

50. Choi SY, Kwon HJ, Ahn GR, et al. Hyaluronic acid microneedle patch for the improvement of crow's feet wrinkles. Dermatol Ther 2017;30(6). https://doi. org/10.1111/dth.12546.

51. Jang M, Baek S, Kang G, et al. Dissolving microneedle with high molecular weight hyaluronic acid to improve skin wrinkles, dermal density and elasticity. Int J Cosmet Sci 2020;42(3):302–9.

52. Searle T, Ali FR, Al-Niaimi F. The versatility of azelaic acid in dermatology. J Dermatol Treat 2022;33: 722–32.

53. Woolery-Lloyd HC, Keri J, Doig S. Retinoids and azelaic acid to treat acne and hyperpigmentation in skin of color. J Drugs Dermatol JDD 2013;12:434–7.

54. Nazzaro-Porro M. The Depigmenting Effect of Azelaic Acid. Arch Dermatol 1990;126:1649.

55. Zaid AN, Al Ramahi R. Depigmentation and Anti-aging Treatment by Natural Molecules. CPD 2019; 25:2292–312.

56. Yamamoto Y, Uede K, Yonei N, et al. Effects of alpha-hydroxy acids on the human skin of Japanese

subjects: The rationale for chemical peeling. J Dermatol 2006;33:16–22.

57. Sharad J. Glycolic acid peel therapy - a current review. Clin Cosmet Invest Dermatol 2013;6:281–8.

58. Babilas P, Knie U, Abels C. Cosmetic and dermatologic use of alpha hydroxy acids: AHA in dermatology. JDDG J der Deutschen Dermatol Gesellschaft 2012; 10:488–91.

59. O'Connor AA, Lowe PM, Shumack S, et al. Chemical peels: A review of current practice. Australas J Dermatol 2018;59:171–81.

60. Kim W-S. Efficacy and safety of a new superficial chemical peel using alpha-hydroxy acid, vitamin C and oxygen for melasma. J Cosmet Laser Ther 2013;15:21–4.

61. Kessler E, Flanagan K, Chia C, et al. Comparison of α- and β-Hydroxy Acid Chemical Peels in the Treatment of Mild to Moderately Severe Facial Acne Vulgaris: Comparison of α- and β-hydroxy acid chemical peels. Dermatol Surg 2007;34:45–51.

62. Oresajo C, Yatskayer M, Hansenne I. Clinical tolerance and efficacy of capryloyl salicylic acid peel compared to a glycolic acid peel in subjects with fine lines/wrinkles and hyperpigmented skin. J Cosmet Dermatol 2008;7:259–62.

63. Arif T. Salicylic acid as a peeling agent: a comprehensive review. Clin Cosmet Invest Dermatol 2015; 8:455–61.

64. Kligman D, Kligman AM. Salicylic Acid Peels for the Treatment of Photoaging. Dermatol Surg 1998;24: 325–8.

65. Garg VK, Sinha S, Sarkar R. Glycolic Acid Peels Versus Salicylic-Mandelic Acid Peels in Active Acne Vulgaris and Post-Acne Scarring and Hyperpigmentation: A Comparative Study. Dermatol Surg 2009;35:59–65.

66. Sarkar R, Garg V, Bansal S, et al. Comparative Evaluation of Efficacy and Tolerability of Glycolic Acid, Salicylic Mandelic Acid, and Phytic Acid Combination Peels in Melasma. Dermatol Surg 2016;42: 384–91.

67. Wójcik A, Kubiak M, Rotsztejn H. Influence of azelaic and mandelic acid peels on sebum secretion in ageing women. pdia 2013;3:140–5.

68. Monheit GD. The Jessner's + TCA Peel: A Medium-Depth Chemical Peel. J Dermatol Surg Oncol 1989; 15:945–50.

69. Lee G-Y, Kim H-J, Whang K-K. The Effect of Combination Treatment of the Recalcitrant Pigmentary Disorders with Pigmented Laser and Chemical Peeling. Dermatol Surg 2002;28:1120–3.

70. Lee KC, Wambier CG, Soon SL, et al. Basic chemical peeling: Superficial and medium-depth peels. J Am Acad Dermatol 2019;81(2):313–24.

71. Yamamoto Y, Uede K, Ohtani T, et al. Different apoptotic patterns observed in tissues damaged

by phenol and TCA peels. J Dermatol Sci Suppl 2006;2:S75–81.

72. Kimura A, Kanazawa N, Li HJ, et al. Influence of chemical peeling on the skin stress response system: Influence of chemical peeling on the skin stress response system. Exp Dermatol 2012;21:8–10.

73. Kontochristopoulos G, Platsidaki E. Chemical peels in active acne and acne scars. Clin Dermatol 2017;35:179–82.

74. Park J-H, Choi Y-D, Kim S-W, et al. Effectiveness of modified phenol peel (Exoderm) on facial wrinkles, acne scars and other skin problems of Asian patients. J Dermatol 2007;34:17–24.

75. Camacho FM. Medium-depth and deep chemical peels. J Cosmet Dermatol 2005;4:117–28.

76. Soon SL, Wambier CG, Rullan PR, et al. International Peeling Society; International Peeling Society. Phenol-Croton Oil Chemical Peeling Induces Durable Improvement of Constitutional Periorbital Dark Circles. Dermatol Surg 2023. https://doi.org/10.1097/DSS.0000000000003708.

77. Tierney EP, Eisen RF, Hanke CW. Fractionated CO2 laser skin rejuvenation: Fractionated CO2 laser skin rejuvenation. Dermatol Ther 2011;24:41–53.

78. Goldman A, Goldust M, Wollina U. Periorbital Hyperpigmentation—Dark Circles under the Eyes; Treatment Suggestions and Combining Procedures. Cosmetics 2021;8:26.

79. Khatri KA, Ross V, Grevelink JM, et al. Comparison of Erbium:YAG and Carbon Dioxide Lasers in Resurfacing of Facial Rhytides. Arch Dermatol 1999;135.

80. Gendler E. Treatment of periorbital hyperpigmentation. Aesthetic Surg J 2005;25:618–24.

81. Fromage G. Microneedling: mechanism of action and indications. Journal of Aesthetic Nursing 2021; 10:144–6.

82. Alster TS, Graham PM. Microneedling: A Review and Practical Guide. Dermatol Surg 2018;44:397–404.

83. Wu SZ, Muddasani S, Alam M. A Systematic Review of the Efficacy and Safety of Microneedling in the Treatment of Melasma. Dermatol Surg 2020;46:1636–41.

84. Singh A, Yadav S. Microneedling: advances and widening horizons. Indian Dermatol Online J 2016; 7:244–54.

85. Naik MN, Honavar SG, Das S, et al. Blepharoplasty: an overview. J Cutan Aesthetic Surg 2009;2:6–11.

86. Paul MD. The evolution of the brow lift in aesthetic plastic surgery. Plast Reconstr Surg 2001;108: 1409–24.

87. Klein AW. Botox for the eyes and eyebrows. Dermatol Clin 2004;22:145–9.

88. Ascher B, Talarico S, Cassuto D, et al. International consensus recommendations on the aesthetic usage of botulinum toxin type A (Speywood Unit) - part II: wrinkles on the middle and lower face, neck and chest: Consensus on lower facial wrinkles treatment with BoNT-A. J Eur Acad Dermatol Venereol 2010;24:1285–95.

89. DeFatta RJ, Williams EF. Fat Transfer in Conjunction with Facial Rejuvenation Procedures. Facial Plastic Surgery Clinics of North America 2008;16:383–90.

90. Brandt FS, Cazzaniga A. Hyaluronic Acid Fillers: Restylane and Perlane. Facial Plastic Surgery Clinics of North America 2007;15:63–76.

91. Gutowski KA. Hyaluronic Acid Fillers. Clin Plast Surg 2016;43:489–96.

Expanding Treatment Indications Beyond the Tear Trough Defect

The G-Point Lift Technique to Address the Entire Eyelid-Cheek Junction

Francesco P. Bernardini, MD[a], Brent Skippen, MD[b,c],*

KEYWORDS

• Tear trough • Filler • Tear trough defect

KEY POINTS

- The authors have developed a more anatomic approach to the infraorbital region, which has led to recognition of a specific anatomic area, defined previously as the aesthetic "G-point."
- Knowledge of the anatomy of the infraorbital region is key to understanding the extent of the clinically visible defect and the underlying structures involved to achieve reliable and reproducible results.
- By shifting attention away from the tear trough itself and applying a surgical approach to aesthetic medicine, one can offer more natural and complete results while at the same time minimizing the risk of undesired side effects and complications.

INTRODUCTION

Knowledge of the anatomy of the infraorbital region is key to understanding the full extent of clinically visible infraorbital defects and the underlying structures involved to achieve optimal aesthetic results. Until recently, most injectors have focused solely on treatment of the tear trough defect with hyaluronic acid fillers to improve the hollowed appearance of this limited, yet relevant area. The most popular treatment consists of a direct tear trough injection, using either a needle or cannula injection technique. However, this direct, "fill-the-hole" approach is flawed by inconsistent results and by somewhat high risks of aesthetic complications.

In a cadaveric study by Cotofana and coworkers,[1] the concept of the surface volume coefficient (SVC) was introduced, a novel parameter used to describe the effectiveness of each facial fat compartment when applying volumizing treatments. The authors of that particular study identified the suborbicularis oculi fat (SOOF) compartment as the most effectively treated facial fat compartment because 95% of injected products in that region are translated into surface projection. The deep medial cheek fat compartment was instead observed to have an SVC of 26%, which indicates that 74% of the injected product fails to translate into surface projection. The concept of a "line of ligaments" was recently introduced by Casabona and colleagues.[2] This imaginary line is the connecting trajectory between the four major facial ligaments:

1. The temporal ligamentous adhesion (temple, upper face)

Funding: None applicable.
[a] Oculoplastica Bernardini, Villa Montallegro, Via Monte Zovetto, 27, 16145 Geneova, Italy; [b] Wagga Wagga NSW 2650, Australia; [c] UNSW Medical School
* Corresponding author. 36 Docker Street, Wagga Wagga 2650, Australia.
E-mail address: brentskippen@gmail.com

Dermatol Clin 42 (2024) 89–95
https://doi.org/10.1016/j.det.2023.06.012

derm.theclinics.com

2. The lateral orbital thickening (periorbital, upper/middle face)
3. The zygomatic ligament (zygomatic arch, middle face)
4. The mandibular ligament (jawline, lower face)

This line of ligaments concept separates the face into a medial and lateral face. Volumizing treatments to the lateral face predominantly result in lifting effects, whereas the same treatments to the medial face result mainly in volumizing effects.[2] Casabona and colleagues[2] used this concept of a line of ligaments in a prospective clinical study and it was reported that the volume needed in the medial midface to achieve a symmetric outcome was significantly reduced if injection points lateral to the line of ligaments were targeted first (lateral injections point should be performed before medial injection points).[2] The authors of that study thus concluded that volumizing treatments to the lateral face reposition the medially located soft tissues, which then require less volume to achieve a symmetric volumizing effect.

Until recently, few injection treatment algorithms for the eyelid-cheek junction were presented that respected the underlying anatomy and made use of such concepts as line of ligaments or SVC. The authors here describe the results of a recently reported injection algorithm, which respects the aforementioned anatomic concepts. This approach takes advantage of the line of ligaments, the SVC, and the G-prime of fillers to better allow the injector to address the entire infraorbital region while minimizing the amount of direct filler injections in the tear trough itself. The first author has previously reported a series of 163 patients from his private practice (FPB), in all cases aiming to first restore the position of the orbicularis retaining ligament (ORL) before then recontouring the inferior orbital rim.[3]

RELEVANT ANATOMY OF THE INFRAORBITAL REGION

Knowledge of the anatomy of the infraorbital region is essential to understand the extent of the clinically visible defect and the underlying structures involved to achieve good results. The so-called "tear-trough" represents only about one-third of the entire infraorbital hollow; it becomes apparent that limiting efforts to this defect only significantly reduces the likelihood of achieving a full aesthetic restoration. The ORL and tear-trough ligaments are two wide structures tightly attached to the anterior face of the maxilla that separate the SOOF from the overlying infraorbital fat.

The surgical experience of the authors has proven that lifting these two ligaments requires complete sharp dissection. This explains why attempts to elevate the ligaments by means of direct filler injection is difficult if not impossible without injecting too much product. In fact, direct injection with a needle on the periosteum of the tear trough defect as advocated by many injectors may push the filler on each side of the ligament, accentuating the defect and predisposing to more potential complications.

INTRODUCING THE G-POINT CONCEPT

The authors understand that as surgeons, an almost complete correction of infraorbital hollowing, eyelid bags, skin laxity and eyelid position is achieved by means of a gentle lateral pull of the orbicularis muscle. As injectors, the authors also understand that the same lateral lift principles have also proven effective in medical lifting, provided one takes advantage of the different G-prime of fillers. This important point, demonstrated in **Fig. 1**, is called the "aesthetic G-point" because it combines a strategic anatomic area with the filler's own G-prime.

DEFINING TREATMENT GOALS

When examining a potential candidate for noninvasive as opposed to surgical treatment, it is always normal practice to routinely dedicate an appropriate amount of time to analyzing the defect at hand and then determine the best treatment plan, respecting the goals in each individual patient to restore a youthfully smoother eyelid-cheek junction. Based on these findings, instead of considering the void of the tear trough as the only goal of filler treatment, the treatment plan is further personalized, including choosing the best products for that patient and the volume of filler in different areas needed to achieve a good result.

In the previous reported study of the senior author (FPB), the desired aesthetic outcome was assessed by the treating physician and by the patient with the following parameters evaluated before and after filler treatment[3]:

- Severity of tear trough/medial infraorbital hollowing as assessed on a five-point Likert scale with 0 = none, 1 = mild, 2 = moderate, 3 = severe, and 4 = very severe
- Severity of palpebromalar groove/lateral infraorbital hollowing as assessed on a five-point Likert scale with 0 = none, 1 = mild, 2 = moderate, 3 = severe, and 4 = very severe
- Severity of hollowing of the entire lid-cheek junction as assessed on a five-point Likert

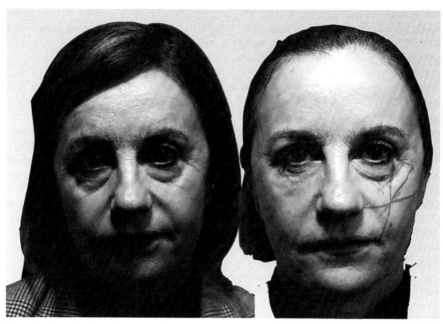

Fig. 1. Finding the G-point in each patient by drawing lines on the patient before treatment is a preparatory moment comparable with surgery, which helps to achieve reproducible and symmetric results in each patient. The G-point is higher and lateral compared with the apex of the malar eminence, located in the lateral SOOF, and lateral to the line of ligaments; therefore it is in the perfect position to exert a lift and stretch effect of the orbital retaining ligament and the deep fascial connections.

scale with 0 = none, 1 = mild, 2 = moderate, 3 = severe, and 4 = very severe
- Global Aesthetic Improvement Scale as assessed on a five-point Likert scale with 0 = much worsened, 1 = worsened, 2 = neutral, 3 = improved, and 4 = much improved

TREATMENT: ALGORITHM PLANNING AND INJECTION TECHNIQUE

In the private practice of the senior author (FPB), the location for product application is marked on the skin surface according to the protocol shown in **Fig. 1**: a connecting line between the inferior aspect of the nasal ala and the tragus, then a connecting line between the lateral canthus and the corner of the mouth, and a connecting line between the intersection of the two lines, and a perpendicular line connecting to the lateral canthus. This dermal location was termed the "G-point," because it combines the G-prime effect, which is maximized in a specific starting point (see **Fig. 1**).

A dermal access puncture is performed with a 21G needle (TSK Laboratory) 1 cm superolateral to the midportion of the nasolabial sulcus. A 22G 50-mm blunt-tip cannula (Dermasculpt) is introduced into the superficial nasolabial fat compartment and advanced in the direction of the

G-point. After the level of the infraorbital foramen is passed, the cannula is introduced deeper into the supraperiosteal plane. This "first-superficial-then-deep" cannula advancement technique ensured that the infraorbital neurovascular structures and the angular vein were both crossed superficially. The correct positioning of the tip of the cannula was digitally controlled and ensured that it corresponded to the lateral aspect of the SOOF and that it was also located lateral to the line of ligaments.[2] In the next step, the cannula is retracted (without exiting the facial soft tissues) and readvanced cranially in the midpupillary line. Three serial bolus injections are then performed in the supraperiosteal plane targeting the upper/middle/lower aspects of the medial SOOF.

Subsequently, the cannula is retracted and readvanced cranially following the "first-superficial-then-deep" approach positioning another supraperiosteal bolus in the palpebromalar groove, inferior to the ORL at the level of the lateral canthus, and another bolus in the supraperiosteal plane in the tear trough. Thus, a total of six boluses of soft tissue filler of high viscoelastic characteristics were positioned in the supraperiosteal plane using one single dermal access puncture. In the following step, the contour between the cheek and the lower eyelid was addressed. Dermal access was made by a 23G needle (TSK Laboratory) in the dermal location of the G-point. A 25G 50-mm blunt-tip cannula (TSK Laboratory) was introduced into the SOOF without establishing bone contact. The cannula was advance medially deep to orbicularis oculi muscle and superior to the ORL. During retrograde movement, small amounts of soft tissue filler (low viscoelastic characteristics) were injected.

Initially, macroboluses (0.1 mL) of a high G-prime filler (RHA4 [Teoxane]) were used with a high G-prime filler injected deeply at the G-point to provide a lifting effect and subsequently at the apex of the V-deformity of the lower eyelid to provide central support. Subsequently, microboluses (0.02–0.03 mL) of a dedicated low G-prime filler, (Redensity II [Teoxane]), were injected along the entire lower eyelid delivered in a bridging technique. Results were determined by objective analysis, comparing preprocedure and postprocedure photographs taken 1 month after the filler injection using a four-point grading scale (where 0* = worsened, 1* = unchanged, 2* = mildly improved, and 4* = greatly improved), and by a subjective, anonymous patient satisfaction questionnaire delivered to each patient by nonmedical assistants at the final follow-up visit, using a similar four-point grading scale.

CLINICAL ASSESSMENT AND MEASUREMENT

Following injection of the G-point (but before injection of the remaining six locations), the distances (measured in millimeters) between the dermal location of the G-point and the inferior aspect of the nasal ala, the corner of the mouth, and the dermal location of the mandibular ligament were assessed and recorded. Additionally, the height of the lower eyelid, that is, the distance between the lower eyelid-cheek junction and the eyelashes, was measured. After treatment completion, improvement of the infraorbital hollowness and the medial midface volume was scored according to the Global Aesthetic Improvement Scale as assessed on a five-point Likert scale with 0 = much worsened, 1 = worsened, 2 = neutral, 3 = improved, and 4 = much improved. The scoring was conducted 6 months after the final

injection and was scored by the patient and by the treating physician separately. Treatment results are shown in **Figs. 2–6**.

DISCUSSION

The effectiveness of the G-point lift is explained by its anatomy: the G-point lies in the most lateral part of the infraorbital region, superolateral to the ORL. The ORL expands laterally to the lateral canthal region to form the lateral orbital thickening, while inferior to the ORL, the zygomatic-cutaneous ligament (ZCL) runs transversely across the malar region. The ZCL (inferiorly) and the ORL (superiorly) form the boundaries of the SOOF and of the fat within the prezygomatic space, which is located deep to the SOOF. Both ligaments (ORL and ZCL) are anchored to the periosteum deep to the orbicularis oculi muscle and lifting their periosteal insertion by means of direct injection is almost impossible without the release of this attachment; however, their dermal connections, visible on the skin surface, are more easily stretched.

The orientation of the ORL and the ZCL change with age and the related soft tissue descent. This orientation of the ligaments changes from more horizontal when younger to more vertical when older. By influencing the orientation of those ligaments with filler treatment, the signs of facial aging might be reduced. Soft tissue filler injected directly below the ORL in patients with a clinical presentation of tear trough and palpebromalar groove hollowing, in the authors' experience, reorients those ligaments and reduces the visible signs of facial aging.

The authors believe that the G-point lift injection is an effective technique because of the anatomic location of the G-point posterior and lateral to the line of ligaments, a position where the dermal adhesion of the ligament is more easily stretched. Injecting a macrobolus of a high G-prime filler, such as Teoxane RHA4, is the first step of this technique, aimed at providing effective stretching of the dermal adhesion of the ORL and ZCL.[3] The second step (contouring phase) is then focused on recontouring of the inferior orbital rim.[3] This step involves

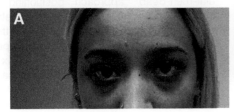
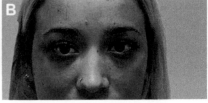

Fig. 2. Clinical photographs of before (*A*) and after (*B*) G-point lifting treatment in a 27-year-old woman showing significant improvement in patient appearance by effacing the eyelid-cheek junction with improvement of the orbitomalar hollow and eyelid bags.

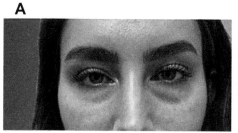
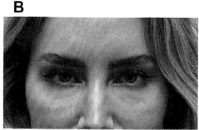

Fig. 3. Clinical photographs of before (*A*) and 1 week after (*B*) G-point lifting treatment in a 34-year-old woman showing significant improvement in patient appearance by effacing the eyelid-cheek junction with improvement of the eyelid bags.

using a 25-gauge blunt tip cannula using a low G-prime filler, such as Teoxane Redensity 2.[3] Both injection steps administer filler right below the ORL and aim to reposition the ORL and, consequently, the midfacial soft tissues.

The G-point lift technique delivers surgical-quality results using a noninvasive approach. The same concept is applied to lower blepharoplasty in the authors' practice; as surgeons, complete lower eyelid rejuvenation is achieved by combining orbicularis suspension performed at the G-point with central eyelid support provided by fat transposition associated with skin tightening.

This surgical concept can be applied to noninvasive treatment of the lower eyelid, taking advantage of different filler rheology features, mainly their G-prime. The surgical habit of preoperative preparatory markings was also applied to the authors' noninvasive treatments; combining one drawing with another has confirmed the existence of the G-point as a common specific point of maximal lifting effect, which maximizes the effect of surgical and nonsurgical approaches equally. As injectors, a strong G-prime filler, delivered in macroboluses of 0.1 mL used at the G-point achieves an eyelid lifting effect; when placed centrally, it provided similar eyelid support as that provided by surgical fat transposition. A low G-prime filler, delivered in microboluses of

0.02 mL, provides smoothing of the transitions at the medial eyelid and also skin tightening. As both surgeons and injectors, the authors have recognized the existence of a common distinct anatomic point with powerful indirect effects, which makes the treatment simpler, more effective, and more reproducible and even requires less direct treatment. A stronger lift is achieved by injecting initially at the G-point, which simultaneously improves the tear trough indirectly, therefore needing a much lesser volume of direct tear trough filler injection.

A strength of the authors' conclusions lies in the large sample size of 163 patients in the previously mentioned study.[3] In that recently published series of 163 patients, mild early edema was observed in 84% of patients and moderate early edema in 7.4% of patients. In all patients, early edema, regardless of severity, resolved fully within 14 days of onset.[3] Patients in the same study who experienced early bruising numbered 27.6%, all of which resolved fully within 7 days of onset.[3] Patients who experienced surface irregularities numbered 6.1%, one of whom required hyaluronidase to dissolve the filler product.[3] Two patients required hyaluronidase injection because of persistent late infraorbital edema.[3]

The pathogenesis of infraorbital edema following filler injection has been explained by

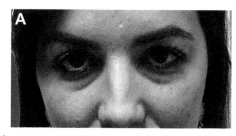
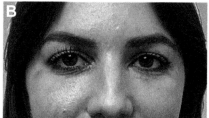

Fig. 4. (*A*) Pretreatment photograph of a 35-year-old woman showing full orbitomalar hollow and tear trough deformity with central and medial intraorbital fat prolapse. (*B*) One week posttreatment photograph showing improvement in the eyelid-cheek junction, eyelid shortening, cheek elevation with improvement of the orbitomalar hollow, and eyelid bags.

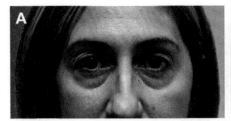
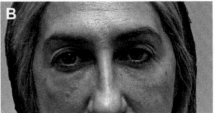

Fig. 5. Clinical photographs of before (*A*) and 1 week after (*B*) G-point lifting treatment in a 48-year-old woman showing significant improvement in patient appearance by effacing the eyelid-cheek junction with improvement of the orbitomalar hollow, eyelid bags, and skin laxity.

the effective lymphatic drainage of the SOOF region.[4] The lymphatic outflow in this region is directed laterally and does not follow the angular vein. Injecting a high G-prime product might impair the lymphatic outflow, which could cause the observed rate of edema. Bruising was attributed in the Cotofana study to the presence of the plethora of arteries and veins located in the infraorbital area.[5]

The injection technique that was used comprised a total of six bolus injections (22G cannula) and one retrograde fanning injection (25G cannula). A blunt-tip cannula technique was used for all seven targeted locations. The cannula advancement of this technique is nonlinear and requires a certain degree of anatomic knowledge. The cannula is first introduced into the superficial fatty layer and, following passage of the infraorbital neurovascular bundle and the angular vein, the cannula is redirected deeper toward the supraperiosteal plane. This "first-superficial-then-deep" cannula advancement ensures that structures at risk for intravascular product placement, such as the infraorbital artery, the zygomaticofacial artery, the transverse facial artery or the angular vein, are respected. These structures are crossed by the cannula superficially, whereas product placement is performed in the supraperiosteal plane. The selected locations for product placement are in line with current anatomic concepts: the line of ligaments and the SVC.

The location of the first bolus injection was termed the G-point. This location corresponds to the lateral boundary of the lateral SOOF, which is located at or lateral to the line of ligaments. To control for proper product placement, digital control of the noninjecting hand is performed during cannula advancement. Once the tip of the cannula reaches the desired location the first (of six in total) bolus injections are performed. In a previously reported study,[6] product was injected lateral to the line of ligaments (the G-point), but near enough to not lose efficacy; this resulted in an increase in midfacial distances between the dermal location of the G-point and the jawline, the corner of the mouth, and the nasal ala in a statistically significant magnitude.

The magnitude of facial soft tissue repositioning in previously reported studies was majorly determined by the high effectiveness of the SOOF, when evaluated by the SVC.[6] The SVC is used as a measure of effectiveness because it is calculated by the ratio between the change in surface volume projection and the injected volume.[1] For the SOOF the SVC is reported as being 93% at 0.5 mL and 95% at 1.0 mL; this is the highest SVC of all measured facial fat compartments (superficial and deep).[1] The described injection algorithm resulted in the repositioning of the midfacial soft tissues, which was additionally confirmed by the reduction of the measured lower eyelid height. The height of the lower eyelid was determined as the distance between the lower eyelid-cheek junction and the eyelashes.

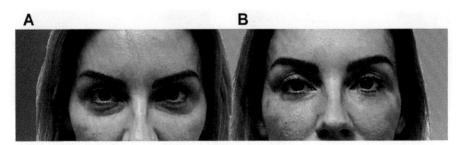

Fig. 6. Clinical photographs of before (*A*) and after (*B*) G-point lifting treatment in a 38-year-old woman showing significant improvement in patient appearance by effacing the eyelid-cheek junction with improvement of the orbitomalar hollow and eyelid bags.

SUMMARY

By shifting attention away from the tear trough itself and also applying a surgical approach to aesthetic medicine, one can begin to offer more natural and complete results while at the same time minimizing the risk of side effects and complications. The detailed cannula injection-based two-step algorithm uses the anatomic concepts of a line of ligaments and SVC and positions the product in the supraperiosteal plane. The initial step aims at restoring the position of the orbital retaining ligament before then directly recontouring the inferior orbital rim. In this way, less direct treatment is required. The results are proof that by using these novel anatomic concepts, a small mean amount of high G-prime soft tissue filler injected in the lateral SOOF (the G-point) can change midfacial distances significantly.

CLINICS CARE POINTS

- The G-point lift injection is an effective 2 step technique because of the anatomic location of the G-point posterior and lateral to the line of ligaments.
- The first step uses a high G-prime filler to provide effective stretching of the dermal adhesion of the ORL and ZCL ligaments.
- The second step uses a low G-prime filler to recontour of the inferior orbital rim.
- Pitfalls:- The "first-superficial-then-deep" cannula advancement technique requires a certain degree of anatomic knowledge.

DISCLOSURE

The authors have no conflicts of interest to disclose.

REFERENCES

1. Cotofana S, Koban KC, Konstantin F, et al. The surface-volume-coefficient of the superficial and deep facial fat compartments: a cadaveric 3D volumetric analysis. Plast Reconstr Surg 2019;143(6): 1605–13.

2. Casabona G, Frank K, Koban KC, et al. Lifting vs volumizing: the difference in facial minimally invasive procedures when respecting the line of ligaments. J Cosmet Dermatol 2019;18(5): 1237–43.

3. Bernardini FP, Casabona G, Alfertshofer MG, et al. Soft tissue filler augmentation of the orbicularis retaining ligament to improve the lid-cheek junction. J Cosmet Dermatol 2021;20(11): 3446–53.

4. Cotofana S, Steinke H, Schlattau A, et al. The anatomy of the facial vein: implications for plastic, reconstructive, and aesthetic procedures. Plast Reconstr Surg 2017;139(6):1346–53.

5. Cotofana S, Lachman N. Arteries of the face and their relevance for minimally invasive facial procedures: an anatomical review. Plast Reconstr Surg 2019;143(2): 416–26.

6. Casabona G, Bernardini FP, Skippen B, et al. How to best utilize the line of ligaments and the surface volume coefficient in facial soft tissue filler injections. J Cosmet Dermatol 2019;00:1–9.

Revisiting the Ligament Line of the Face
A New Understanding for Filling the Fixed and Mobile Face

Andre Braz, MD[a], Eliandre Palermo, MD[b], Maria Claudia Issa, MD, PhD[c],*

KEYWORDS

- Ligament line • Mobile face • Fixed face • Cosmetic procedures • Fillers • Hyaluronic acid
- Calcium hydroxyapatite • Poly-L- Lactic acid

KEY POINTS

- To understand the facial anatomy and the facial anatomy of aging, it is necessary to interpret the retaining ligaments as anatomic landmarks.
- In recent years, with remarkable advances in surgical treatments and facial aesthetics procedures, the importance of retaining ligaments, described by Mendelson and Stuzin as anatomic landmarks, has become essential to understand facial anatomy in a 3-dimensional way.
- The ligaments are usually positioned in fixed anatomic locations, and their superficial extensions form the subcutaneous septa that permeate the facial fat compartments.

 Video content accompanies this article at http://www.derm.theclinics.com.

INTRODUCTION

To understand the facial anatomy and the facial anatomy of aging, it is necessary to interpret the retaining ligaments as anatomic landmarks. In recent years, with remarkable advances in surgical treatments and facial aesthetics procedures, the importance of retaining ligaments, described by Mendelson and Stuzin as anatomic landmarks, has become essential to understand facial anatomy in a 3-dimensional way.[1–3]

The ligaments function as anchorage points supporting the skin and the subcutaneous tissue, and, together with the superficial musculoaponeurotic system (SMAS) and the cutis retinaculum, contribute to the formation of the furrows and shadows of the face in the aging process. The ligaments are usually positioned in fixed anatomic locations, and their superficial extensions form the subcutaneous septa that permeate the facial fat compartments. Over the years, different descriptions of the retentor ligaments of the face have been published in the literature, and various classifications, locations, and nomenclature systems have been proposed.[4]

The ligament line is an anatomic landmark that divides the face into 2 parts, where the layers are arranged differently anteriorly and posteriorly.[5] Mendelson was one of the first authors to emphasize the functional division of the face by a vertical line of ligaments separating the anterior from the posterior face. He described these ligaments from top to bottom as temporal, lateral orbital, zygomatic, masseteric, and mandibular ligaments.[1] The anterior

[a] Private Clinic, Rua Visc. de Pirajá, 547 - Grupo 801 - Ipanema, Rio de Janeiro - RJ, 22410-900, Brazil; [b] Private Clinic, Av. São Gualter, 1036 - Alto de Pinheiros, São Paulo - SP, 05455-001, Brazil; [c] Associate Professor of Dermatology in the Department of Internal Medicine at Fluminense Federal University, Av. Marquês do Paraná, 303- Centro, Niterói, RJ. CEP:24033-900
* Corresponding author.
E-mail address: mariaissa@id.uff.br

Dermatol Clin 42 (2024) 97–102
https://doi.org/10.1016/j.det.2023.07.006

mobile face is adapted to the mimetic expressions, and the posterior fixed face is represented by the SMAS and the masticatory structures (**Fig. 1**). Anteriorly, the facial layers are oriented obliquely to the skin surface. In contrast, posteriorly, they are parallel to the skin surface. Because of the soft tissue arrangement and the mimetic muscle, filling these different face layers promotes specific effects. When injected anteriorly, it results in a volumizing, whereas laterally, it causes a lifting effect.[6]

THE NEW UNDERSTANDING OF THE FACIAL LIGAMENT LINE

Based on the scientific literature, the authors' clinical experience, and observations during the dissection of fresh frozen cadavers, the authors emphasize 2 crucial questions about the facial ligament line. Is the jowl deformity part of the mobile or fixed face? Is the ligament line a vertical line or an oblique line?

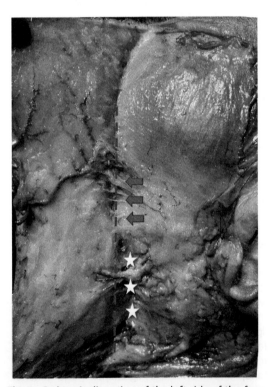

Fig. 1. Cadaveric dissection of the left side of the face exposing the SMAS, superficial temporal fascia with the superficial temporal artery and the temporal fascia (*upper face*), and the parotid masseteric fascia (*middle and low face*). The blue arrows mark the zygomatic ligament. The white stars mark the masseteric ligaments on the anterior border of the masseter muscle (posteriorly to the mandibular ligament). The dashed pink line represents the functional ligament line (fLL).

The anatomy of the jowl and the mandibular ligament were recently reassessed. Unlike previous studies, Minelli and colleagues[7] described that the mandibular ligament is formed by the combined muscular (depressor muscles and platysma) attachments to the mandible and is profoundly located in the subplatysmal layer. It extends from the labiomandibular crease to the anterior border of the masseter (**Fig. 2**A, B). Because of aging, a redundant subcutaneous and dermis develop to form the jowl, which overlies the mandibular ligament to create tissue mobility with considerable variation in position and extension.[8] During jaw opening or smiling, the jowl region moves up and back (Video 1), which justifies questioning the current concept of the oblique line of ligaments that encompasses the mandibular ligament. This virtual oblique line aligned the facial ligaments located immediately lateral to the lateral orbital rim extending from the temporal ligamentous adhesion, lateral orbital thickening, zygomatic ligament, and mandibular ligament.[6] Conversely, this line did not limit the mobile and fixed face functionally, as the low point of this line is anterior to the movable jowl fat.

The authors propose a new approach for this line, renamed the functional ligament line of the face (fLL), in which the lower point is the masseteric ligament and not the mandibular ligament. It functionally divides the fixed face posteriorly to it, obeying the dynamic facial expressions and jowl's movement (**Fig. 2**C, D).

HOW TO CHOOSE FILLERS BASED ON THE FUNCTION LIGAMENT LINE: AUTHORS' EXPERIENCE

Different techniques and fillers are described for facial rejuvenation or beautification. Medical assessment and anatomy are crucial to reach good results and avoid adverse effects. During clinical evaluation, ethnicity, gender, facial shapes, proportions, and asymmetries should be considered.

When treating the face, it is frequently necessary to associate more than one injectable type with different mechanisms of action and rheologic properties because of unique anatomic characteristics of mobile and fixed areas, which fLL limits (**Fig. 3**). This border functionally shares the injectables according to their physicochemical characteristics.

According to the clinical assessment, hyaluronic acid (HA) gels with moderate-high elasticity and cohesivity are indicated for lifting and structuring. They are applied in the middle and lower face anteriorly and posteriorly to the fLL. Gels with moderate-high elasticity or large particles are

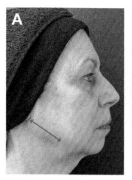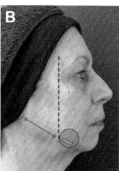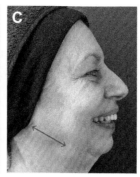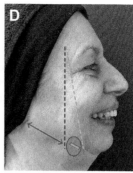

Fig. 2. (A–D) Aged patient showing evident jowl fat in the lower face (profile picture). (A, B) Mandibular line with evident jowl fat in the static position. The oblique (*dashed green line*) represents the ligament line (LL) ending anteriorly to the jowl fat (JF). The straight line (*dashed pink line*) represents the fLL, which ends posteriorly to the JF. The pink arrow delimits the fixed face. The blue line represents the mandibular ligament (ML). The orange circle represents the jowl fat. (C, D) The patient showed jowl fat modification (*orange circle*) during smiling without changing the fLL or the fixed face (*pink arrow*).

used for volumizing the midface anteriorly to the fLL. HA gels with low-moderate elasticity and cohesivity are used for refining the fixed and mobile face in the upper, middle, and lower face.

The biostimulating agents, such as calcium hydroxyapatite (CaHA) or poly-ʟ- lactic acid (PLLA), induce a lifting effect and improve skin quality but cannot be used to volumize or refine and

should be applied posteriorly to the fLL. For this reason, they are commonly applied in association with HA gels in the same session.

A new generation of fillers combines HA gel with different biostimulating agents in the same composition. An innovative composite matrix of CaHA in the gel of HA, available in Brazil and many other countries, has a specific manufacturing process with unique rheologic characteristics with high elasticity, different from manually mixing HA gel and CaHA in a syringe before a procedure. Therefore, it is indicated to be applied in the middle and lower face to promote structure and lift.

Summing up, HA gels can be applied anteriorly and posteriorly to the fLL in the upper, middle, and lower face, depending on their rheologic properties and the patient assessment. Biostimulating agent is indicated to be applied posteriorly to the fLL in the upper, middle, and lower face, and the composite matrix in the middle and lower face posteriorly to the fLL.

INJECTABLES' RHEOLOGIC PROPERTIES AND THEIR RELATION TO THE FUNCTIONAL LIGAMENT LINE AND THE ANATOMIC LAYER

HA gel is applied anteriorly and posteriorly to the fLL in the upper face in the temporal, forehead, and eyebrow (retro-orbicularis oculus fat), preferentially using a 22G cannula. In the temporal region, HA gel fillers with low-moderate elasticity and cohesivity with small-intermediate particle size are indicated to fill and lift. They can be applied on the subcutaneous layer above the superficial temporal fascia (STF) (**Fig. 4**A) or between the STF and the superficial layer of the deep temporal fascia (**Fig. 4**B). In the supraperiosteal layer, HA with high elasticity can be applied with a

Fig. 3. The fLL that functionally divides the fixed face posteriorly to it, obeying the dynamic facial expressions.

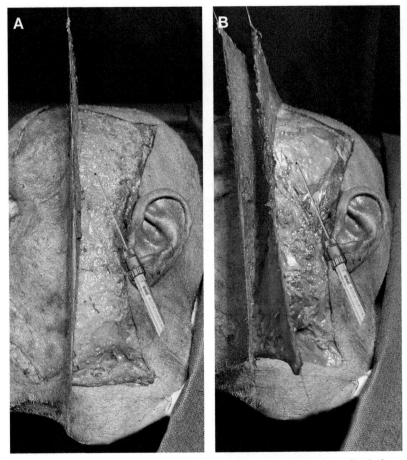

Fig. 4. In the temporal region, they (fillers) can be applied on the subcutaneous layer (SCL) above the STF (*A*) or between the STF and the superficial layer of the deep temporal fascia (DTF) (*B*).

needle (**Fig. 5**). Biostimulating agents should be applied in the superficial fat above the STF, posteriorly to the fLL. The HA gel should be applied in the supraperiosteal layer on the forehead. Ultrasound to guide the procedures in the upper face is indicated to increase safety.

In the middle face, HA gels with moderate-high elasticity and cohesivity with intermediate-large particle size are indicated to promote lifting in the lateral zygoma and support and volume in the deep pyriform space, malar area, malar prominence, and medial zygoma anteriorly to the fLL. They should be applied preferentially in deep fat compartments or supraperiosteal with a 22G cannula (**Fig. 6**). Gel with low-moderate elasticity and cohesivity with small-intermediate particle size is indicated for refinement, applied in the superficial fat with a 22G cannula in the malar region, the nasolabial fold, and infrazygoma (**Fig. 7**). The same gel for refinement treats the eyelid-cheek junction, but the correct anatomic layer is under the orbicularis oculi muscle. The nose is a complex

region for filling, and the HA gel should present moderate-high elasticity and moderate-high cohesivity. It is preferentially applied with a 22G cannula, but needles are also possible. The supraperiosteal and supraperichondrial are the safest layers, but ultrasound guidance is appreciated. The composite matrix of CaHA in the gel of HA should be applied posteriorly to the fLL with a 22G cannula in the subcutaneous layer in the lateral and infrazygoma.

In the lower face, posteriorly to the fLL, HA gels with high elasticity are used to structure and define the jawline (**Fig. 8**). They should be applied in the subcutaneous layer in the mandibular ramus, angle, and body using a 22G cannula. Needles can also be used for supraperiosteal application in the angle. The same gel can be applied in the pre-jowl and the mental area, both in superficial and deep fat compartments. Gel with low-moderate elasticity and cohesivity with small-intermediate particle size is indicated for refinement, applied in a subcutaneous layer in the

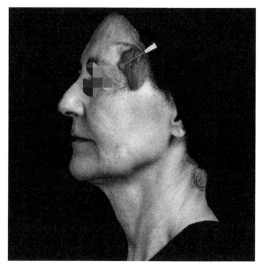

Fig. 5. In the temporal region HA filler with high elasticity can be applied supraperiosteal with a needle.

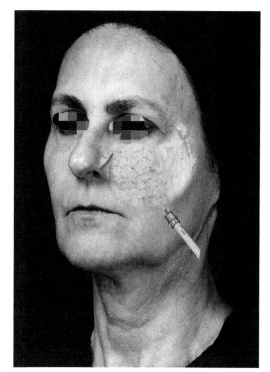

Fig. 7. In the middle face, gel with low-moderate elasticity and cohesivity with small-intermediate particle size is indicated for refinement, applied in the superficial fat with a 22G cannula in the malar region.

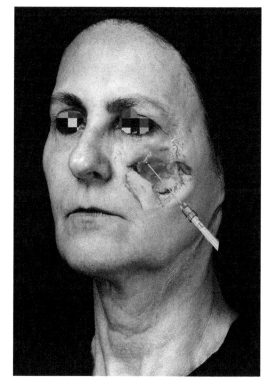

Fig. 6. In the middle face, HA gels should be applied preferentially in deep fat compartments or supraperiosteal with a 22G cannula.

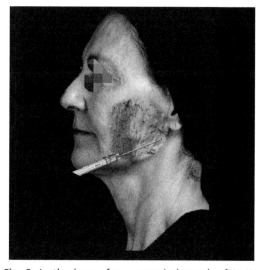

Fig. 8. In the lower face, posteriorly to the fLL, HA gels with high elasticity are used to structure and define the jawline.

perioral area, labio-mental and labio-mandibular folds. The same HA gel can be used in the lips above and under the orbicularis oris muscle. The composite matrix of CaHA in a gel of HA should be applied posteriorly to the fLL with a 22G cannula in the subcutaneous layer in the mandibular ramus, angle, and body.

SUMMARY

Over time, different approaches to the ligament line of the face were reported. Vertical or oblique, it was described to divide the face into anterior mobile and posterior fixed anatomically. This line has been used to guide cosmetic procedures due to differences in soft tissue arrangement and mimetic muscles. Despite this justification, the previous description of this line virtually linked ligaments from the temporal region until the mandibular line, not obeying the fixed and movable face.

The authors revisited this line, unifying the anatomy structures and facial functionality, and entitled it as fLL.

CLINICS CARE POINTS

- The ligament line is used to guide facial lifting or volumizing procedures.

- The ligament line first described in the literature includes the jowl fat, part of the mobile face.

- The new functional Ligament Line redefined the limit between the fixed and mobile face, excluding the movable jowl fat, guiding the lifting or volumizing procedures properly.

DISCLOSURE

None.

SUPPLEMENTARY DATA

Supplementary data to this article can be found online at https://doi.org/10.1016/j.det.2023.07.006.

REFERENCES

1. Mendelson BC. Facelift anatomy, SMAS, retaining ligaments and facial spaces. In: Aston J, Steinbrech DS, Walden JL, editors. Aesthetic Plastic Surgery. London: Saunders Elsevier; 2009. p. 53–72.

2. Mendelson BC, Wong CH. Chapter 6: Anatomy of the Aging Face. In: Neligan PC, Warren RJ, editors. Plastic surgery. 3rd Edition; Volume 2. Aesthetic New York, NY: Elsevier; 2012. p. 78–92.

3. Stuzin JM, Baker TJ, Gordon HL. The relationship of the superficial and deep facial fascias: relevance to rhytidectomy and aging. Plast Reconstr Surg 1992; 89(3):441–9.

4. Mohammed Alghoul MD, Mark A, Codner MD. Retaining ligaments of the face: review of anatomy and clinical applications. Aesthetic Surg J 2013;33(6):769–82.

5. Cotofana S, Fratila A, Schenck T, et al. The anatomy of the aging face: a review. Facial Plast Surg 2016;32(3): 253–60.

6. Casabona G, Frank K, Koban KC, et al. Lifting vs volumizing—the difference in facial minimally invasive procedures when respecting the line of ligaments. J Cosmet Dermatol 2019;18(5):1237–43.

7. Minelli L, Yang H-M, van der Lei B, et al. The surgical anatomy of the jowl and the mandibular ligament reassessed. Aesth Plast Surg 2023;47:170–8.

8. Braz A, Eduardo CCP. Reshaping the lower face using injectable fillers. Indian J Plast Surg 2020;1–11.

Comparative Clinical and Histomorphologic Evaluation of the Effectiveness of Combined Use of Calcium Hydroxyapatite and Hyaluronic Acid Fillers for Aesthetic Indications

Ya.A. Yutskovskaya, MD[a], Evgeniya Altarovna Kogan, MD[b],
A.Yu. Koroleva, MD[c], Hassan I. Galadari, MD[d],*

KEYWORDS

- Dermal fillers • Hyaluronic acid • Calcium hydroxylapatite • Immunohistochemistry

KEY POINTS

- Fillers, such as hyaluronic acid and calcium hydroxylapatite, can be used to both volumize and stimulate the body's own collagen to a certain degree.
- Combination approach using multiple modalities in specific sequence for the safe and effective treatment of the aging face.
- Simultaneous injection of the studied products is possible from the point of view of safety, but different levels of administration will be more optimal, and provide a more pronounced remodeling effect on the skin.

INTRODUCTION

The age-related changes that we observe on the faces of our patients in the form of wrinkles, folds, creases, changes in the contour of the face, and loss of volume are associated with changes that occur at the levels of all 5 anatomic layers of the face: bone skeleton, ligaments, muscles, adipose tissue, and skin. The work of an aesthetic doctor should consist of the creation of an optimal comprehensive protocol of procedures that are aimed at those problems with a solution that will lead to maximum results in the form of clinical visual improvement, as well as having a therapeutic effect on the soft tissues of the face. In order to achieve naturalness and harmony, it is necessary to smooth out moderately pronounced and deep facial wrinkles and folds, treat the hypertonus of facial muscles, replenish lost volumes, moisturize the skin, and restore its elasticity.

It is important to understand that to achieve such a complex task of facial rejuvenation, combination treatment of technology and soft tissue augmentation with injectable fillers and neuromodulators must be used. The question is when and how to combine such aesthetic interventions

[a] Dermatovenerology and Cosmetology Department, Pacific State Medical University of Health, Moscow, Russian Federation; [b] Department of Anatomic Pathology, Sechenov University, Moscow, Russian Federation; [c] Center for the Treatment of Complications of Professor Yutskovskaya's Clinic, Moscow, Russian Federation; [d] Department of Medicine, College of Medicine and Health Sciences, United Arab Emirates University, Al Ain, UAE
* Corresponding author.
E-mail address: hgaladari@uaeu.ac.ae

Dermatol Clin 42 (2024) 103–111
https://doi.org/10.1016/j.det.2023.06.011

safely and effectively on the face, hands, neck, and decollete.

Hyaluronic acid and calcium hydroxylapatite can help in replenishing lost volume as well as stimulating the dermis to produce new collagen, respectively. Individually these materials have been used for treating facial lipoatrophy, associated with either human immunodeficiency virus or age, or more generally facial soft tissue volume loss.[1–5] The materials have also been approved to create a smoother and/or fuller appearance in the face, including nasolabial folds, cheeks, and lips and for increasing the volume of the back of the hand.[6,7]

Hyaluronic acid has been studied, either for facial treatments or for treatment of atrophic scars, and proved its effectiveness and has a favorable and well-characterized safety profile.[1,2,8] It has become the gold standard that is compared with all dermal filler studies. Calcium hydroxylapatite is the only biodegradable filler that immediately restores lost volume and simultaneously stimulates the production of natural skin collagen to achieve long-term results.[9] It is a versatile injectable implant and a valuable tool for short- and long-term cosmetic and reconstructive treatments. This injectable is often used in conjunction with botulinum toxin as well as other injectables and energy-based devices. Its effectiveness and safety have been also demonstrated in several studies.[10–12]

Combined aesthetic interventions have widespread application in clinical practice, but results are infrequently reported at scientific meetings and in the medical literature, as there are many variables that need to be investigated. Given the complexity of facial aging, expert consensus supports a combination approach using multiple modalities in specific sequence for the safe and effective treatment of the aging face.[13,14]

The aim of this study is to evaluate histomorphologic findings following Belotero Volume (CPM-HA V) (Merz Aesthetics, Raleigh, NC, USA), a hyaluronic acid–based volumizing filler, and compatibility of a combination of CPM-HA V and Radiesse (Merz Aesthetics, Raleigh, NC, USA), a gel consistent of calcium hydroxylapatite microspheres in carboxymethylcellulose vehicle, in 2 patient groups.

MATERIAL AND METHODS
Study Design

This is an open-label, prospective, pilot, randomized, comparative clinical study and immunohistochemical analysis in healthy female volunteers, 35 to 45 years of age with body mass index (BMI) less than 21. Each subject signed the informed consent form to participate in the study. Ethical approval for the study was obtained in accordance with the ethical principles of the declaration of Helsinki and the International Conference on Harmonisation of Good clinical practice December 2019 to July 2020.

Study Participants

In total, 8 female volunteers aged 35 to 45 years with BMI less than 21, who had indications for lower face, neck, and décolleté lifting, participated in the study. All study subjects completed the study.

During the study, the study subjects had one intradermal CPM-HA V injection into integumentary tissues of the periauricular area (subdermal injection) and followed simultaneous subdermal Radiesse injection into the same area.

Eight study subjects met inclusion/exclusion criteria and were randomly assigned to experimental groups with a 1:1 allocation as per a computer-generated randomization schedule into 2 groups: Group I (CPM-HA V injection and followed Radiesse injection in 1 month)—4 subjects and Group II (CPM-HA V injection and simultaneous Radiesse injection)—4 subjects. Subjects were followed-up for 5 months.

Each subject had a case report form that included information on the date and frequency of procedures, gender, age, area of product injection, biopsy area marking, procedure tolerability assessment score, and assessment of any side effects.

Study Treatments

The study was composed of 3 visits.

Volunteers in Group 1 had intradermal CPM-HA V injections into integumentary tissues of the periauricular area (subdermal injection) at stage 1 (D01). The 27 G 19 mm needle is inserted at an angle of 35° to 40° into the dermis. Standard Radiesse was injected intradermally into one's integumentary tissues of the periauricular area (subdermal injection) in a month at stage 2 (M01). The 27 G 19 mm needle is inserted at an angle of 35 to 40° into the dermis.

Volunteers in Group 2 had intradermal CPM-HA V injections into integumentary tissues of the periauricular area (subdermal injection). Then standard Radiesse was injected intradermally into one's integumentary tissues of the periauricular area (subdermal injection). Both injections were performed at stage 1 (D01). The 27 G 19 mm needle is inserted at an angle of 35° to 40° into the dermis.

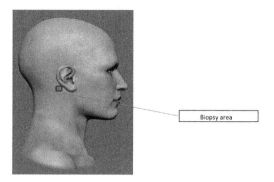

Fig. 1. Punch biopsy area scheme.

Punch biopsy from the treated periauricular area was performed at all 3 visits (**Fig. 1**).

Study Endpoints

Efficacy
As an endpoint the histomorphologic evaluation based on the type I collagen, the type III collagen, and the elastic fibers' analysis using immunohistochemistry test (IHC) in terms of the compatibility of the combination of CPM-HA V and Radiesse was assessed at stage 2 (M01) and at stage 3 (M06) compared with the baseline data.

For the IHC test the patient biopsies samples were fixed in 10% neutral formalin and paraffin embedded. Series of paraffin sections, 4 μm each, were prepared and stained using hematoxylin and eosin, Van Gieson, and Weigert elastic stain. ICH reactions were carried out by antigen retrieval in a retriever according to the standard protocol. Monoclonal anticollagen I antibodies (murine-derived monoclonal antibodies produced by Santa Cruz [sc293182], clone 3G3, dilution 1:100), collagen III (murine-derived monoclonal antibodies produced by Santa Cruz [sc-166316], clone B-4, dilution 1:100), and vascular endothelial growth factor (VEGF) (rabbit polyclonal antibodies produced by Abcam [ab-183100], dilution 1:100) were used. Reactions were performed with positive and negative controls in the absence of primary antibodies.

A comparative analysis of type I and type III collagen, elastin, and other histomorphologic characteristics (presence of an inflammatory reaction, angiogenesis) included 3 zones of the sample (subepithelial, superficial, and deep dermal layers). Staining intensity (on a point-based scale) of samples for histology and immunohistochemistry was assessed using a semiquantitative method. Mild staining corresponded to marker expression of 2 points: moderate—4 points and high—6 points.

Safety
Adverse events were assessed and recorded at each of the 3 visits.

Statistical Analysis

The study was planned to be a pilot, and sample size was not determined. Descriptive statistics are given for each studied parameter. Mann-Whitney test was used to analyze the between-group differences for the study efficacy endpoints. Within the group comparison of the study efficacy endpoints was conducted using Wilcoxon test.

The statistical analysis was performed with the Stata application software (StataCorp, USA) version 14.

RESULTS
Study Population

Eight screened healthy female volunteers met the inclusion/exclusion criteria and were randomized 1:1 into 2 groups. All study subjects completed

Fig. 2. Patients' distribution.

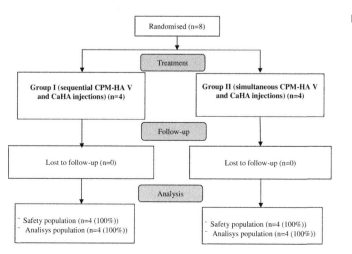

the study without significant protocol deviations. Safety population includes all the patients who received at least one dose of study medications (**Fig. 2**).

All the enrolled subjects were divided into 2 groups:

- Group 1 to 4 patients who received CPM-HA V injection and followed injection of standard Radiesse in a month.
- Group 2 to 4 patients who received CPM-HA V injection and simultaneous injection of standard Radiesse.

Available demographic and clinical data show no difference between the 2 groups before treatment; the 2 groups are comparable in terms of the tested parameters.

Efficacy Outcomes

Histomorphological evaluation of the efficacy
Comparative histology and histochemistry changes Comparative analysis of skin biopsy histomorphology before, 1 month and 5 months after the combined injections of CPM-HA V and Radiesse were performed. Eight punch skin biopsy specimens from the retroauricular area of all 8 study subjects were analyzed.

At the baseline in both groups elastic stain showed no elastic fibers in the subepithelial and superficial layers of the dermis; instead, these were observed as individual fibers within the perivascular and periglandular tissues in the deep dermal layers (0 points).

One month after the single injection of CPM-HA V, Group 1 revealed remodeling of the epidermis due to the accumulation of elastic fibers and an increase in the amount of extracellular matrix. There

are no pathologic changes in the epidermis; the layer did not show any thickening, and there was preserved stratification. Sample evaluation showed no signs of hyperkeratosis. Both papillary and reticular layers of the dermis were not thick and were relatively easy to distinguish. There were multidirectional collagen fibers with a moderate number of slightly unevenly distributed fibroblasts and fibrocytes. The dermis (with hematoxylin and eosin staining and Van Gieson staining) showed extracellular matrix accumulation with the deposition of collagen bundles. There were slightly more vessels (small veins, venules, capillaries, and arterioles) in the dermis compared with stage 1 ($p<0.05$) that revealed lumen enlargement and relatively even distribution of the sample, and their number is similar to those seen at stage 1. Elastic stain revealed elastic fibers (2–4 points) mainly in the superficial and deep dermal layers located around vessels and skin appendages ($p<0.05$).

In Group 2, there was mild remodeling of the dermis due to extracellular matrix accumulation, signs of angiogenesis, and the accumulation of elastic fibers. With hematoxylin and eosin staining and Van Gieson staining, the dermis also revealed deposition of collagen bundles in the extracellular matrix. There were few lymphocytes present in an uneven distribution in the field of view and were typically located in perivascular spaces within the walls of small blood vessels as well as close to some hair follicles. They were not indicative of an inflammatory reaction at the site of filler implantation. There were slightly more vessels (small veins, venules, capillaries, and arterioles) present in the dermis compared with stage 1($p<0.05$). These findings may also be considered morphologic signs of

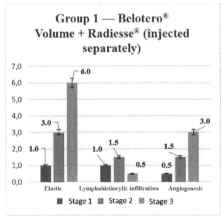
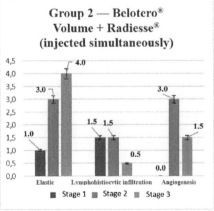

Fig. 3. Comparative analysis of skin biopsy histomorphology before, 1 month and 5 months after the combined injections of CPM-HA V and Radiesse.

Group 1 — Belotero® Volume + Radiesse® (injected separately)

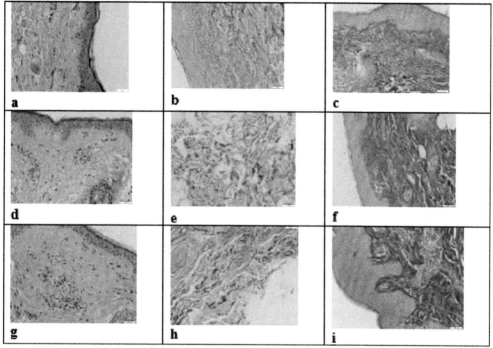

Group 2 — Belotero® Volume + Radiesse® (injected simultaneously)

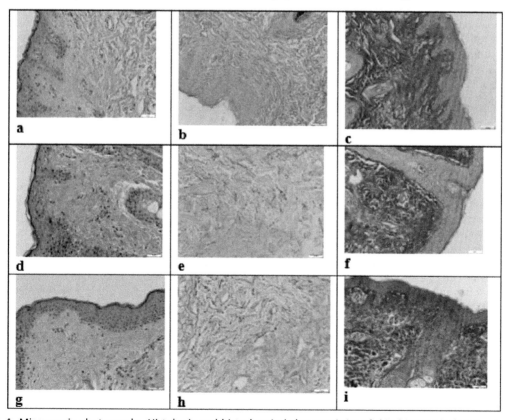

Fig. 4. Microscopic photographs. Histologic and histochemical characteristics of skin biopsies before treatment (A, B, C), 1 month (D, E, F), and 5 months after the combined injections of CPM-HA V and Radiesse (G, H, I). Stains: hematoxylin and eosin (A, D, H), orcein (B, E, H), and Van Gieson picrofuchsin (C, F, I), X 400.

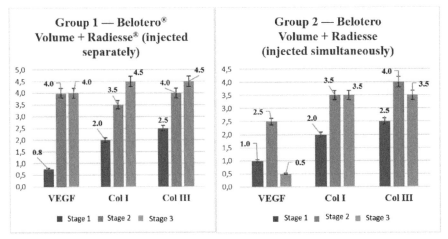

Fig. 5. Comparative analysis of skin biopsy histochemistry before, 1 month, and 5 months after the simultaneous injection of the combination of CPM-HA V and CaHA.

active connective tissue remodeling at the site of dermal filler injection (2–4 points). Elastic stain revealed elastic fibers ($P<0.5$) mainly in the superficial and deep dermal layers located around vessels and skin appendages (2–4 points).

A greater rate of angiogenesis ($p<0.05$) was observed in Group 2, 1 month after the simultaneous injection of CPM-HA V and Radiesse.

Five months after the combined injections of CPM-HA V and Radiesse comparative analysis of skin histomorphology revealed that both products caused remodeling in one's skin, whereas separate injection of CPM-HA V and Radiesse resulted in greater skin remodeling characterized by the following: trend toward ECM accumulation; more pronounced accumulation of elastic fibers ($p<0.05$); enhanced angiogenesis within 4 months after the injection ($p<0.05$).

The results are shown in **Figs. 3** and **4**.

Comparative immunohistochemistry changes In both groups at stage 1 before products injection type I collagen is observed as thin interlacing fibers in the dermis found mainly in the subepithelial and superficial layers. Type III collagen is observed as thicker interlacing fibers of similar location in the dermis and in an amount similar to that of type I collagen: collagen I/III ratio = 1.0. VEGF is observed as cytoplasmic staining in isolated vascular endothelial cells (0–2 points).

A comparative analysis of immunohistochemical characteristics of the tissues following the sequential injections of CPM-HA V and Radiesse as well as simultaneous injections of CPM-HA V and Radiesse showed that these interventions had a remodeling effect on the dermis although the separate injections of CPM-HA V and Radiesse

had a relatively greater effect. This conclusion is supported by more intense type I to III collagen accumulation ($p<0.5$) in the dermis and preservation of the 1:1 ratio as well as intense angiogenesis ($p<0.5$) that provides sustained blood supply to the skin after sequential injections of CPM-HA V and Radiesse performed in Group 1.

The results are shown in **Figs. 5** and **6**.

Safety Outcomes

During the study, no adverse events were reported.

DISCUSSION

The results of this study demonstrate that the injections of the combined injections of CPM-HA V and CaHA lead to histomorphological improvement. A comparative analysis of histomorphological changes in tissues revealed that the products cause remodeling of the skin, with the combined use of CPM-HA V and standard CaHA having a considerable impact on aging and skin remodeling due to ECM accumulation of elastic fibers ($P<0,5$).

Previous studies reported an increase in collagen type III with a gradual equalizing of the ratio toward collagen type I.[11,15] This study, however, showed an increase in the amount of both collagen type I and collagen type III with the same ratio.

According to our results, the sequential injections of CPM-HA V and CaHA had a relatively greater remodeling effect on one's skin compared with the simultaneous injections of CPM-HA V and CaHA. This is confirmed by more intense type I to III collagen accumulation ($p<0.5$) in the dermis and preservation of the 1:1 ratio as well as intense angiogenesis ($p<0.5$) that provides sustained

Group 1 — Belotero® Volume + Radiesse® (injected separately)

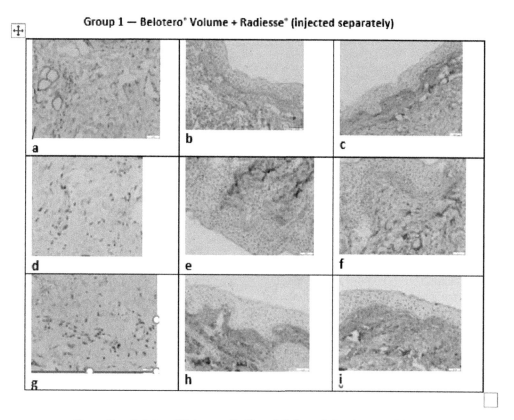

Group 2 — Belotero® Volume + Radiesse® (injected simultaneously)

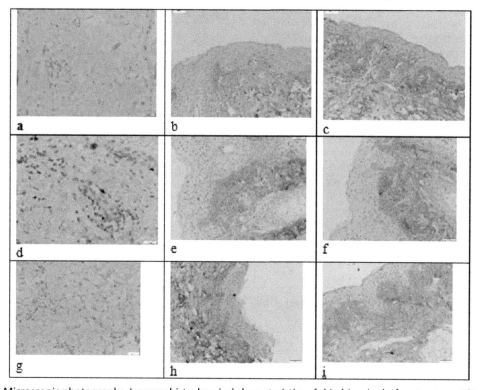

Fig. 6. Microscopic photographs. Immunohistochemical characteristics of skin biopsies before treatment (*A, B, C*), 1 month (*D, E, F*), and 5 months after the combined injections of CPM-HA V and CaHA (*G, H, I*). Immunoperoxidase reactions for VEGF (*A, D, H*), type I collagen (*B, E, H*), and type III collagen (*C, F, I*), Ч 400.

blood supply to the skin after consecutive injections of CPM-HA V and CaHA.

SUMMARY

In conclusion, the data from this randomized, open, prospective, pilot, clinical study correspond to displaying the efficacy in terms of the histomorphological evaluation of the sequential injections of CPM-HA V and CaHA and simultaneous injections of CPM-HA V and CaHA. A comparative analysis of histology and immunohistochemistry of samples following the combined injection of CPM-HA V and CaHA revealed that phased injections of CPM-HA V and CaHA had a greater expected remodeling effect on one's skin compared with simultaneous injection of CPM-HA V and CaHA; this is confirmed by intense elastic fiber formation ($p<0.05$), type I to III collagen accumulation in the dermis ($p<0.05$) with the preserved 1:1 ratio, and intense angiogenesis ($p<0.5$) that provides sustained blood supply to the tissues. There is also evidence that simultaneous injection of CPM-HA V and CaHA at the same level is safe, confirming that there are no histologic and immunohistologic signs of inflammation and disturbance of tissue trophicity.

If we interpret the data obtained regarding clinical practice, we can draw the following conclusion: simultaneous injection of the studied products is possible from the point of view of safety, but different levels of administration will be more optimal, which will provide a more pronounced remodeling effect on the skin.

OTHER INFORMATION

Merz Pharmaceuticals GmbH, Frankfurt am Main, Germany, provided financial support for the manuscript preparation. None of the authors received any financial support for the writing of this article. All listed authors approved the article for submission.

CLINICS CARE POINTS

- Hyaluronic acid and calcium hydroxylapatite may be combined in the same treatment to provide and added benefit.
- Care should be utilized when using calcium hydroxylapatite as, unlike hyaluronic acid, may not dissolve with hyaluronidase.
- Combination therapy is key to tackle the different signs of ageing.

DISCLOSURE

The authors have no conflicts of interest when writing this author.

REFERENCES

1. Micheels P, Vandeputte J, Kravtsov M. Treatment of Age-related Mid-face Atrophy by Injection of Cohesive Polydensified Matrix Hyaluronic Acid Volumizer. J Clin Aesthet Dermatol 2015;8(3):28–34.
2. Becker M, Balagué N, Montet X, et al. Hyaluronic Acid Filler in HIV-Associated Facial Lipoatrophy: Evaluation of Tissue Distribution and Morphology with MRI. Dermatology 2015;230(4):367–74.
3. Silvers SL, Eviatar JA, Echavez MI, et al. Prospective, open-label, 18-month trial of calcium hydroxylapatite (Radiesse) for facial soft-tissue augmentation in patients with human immunodeficiency virusassociated lipoatrophy: one-year durability. Plast Reconstr Surg 2006;118(3 Suppl):34S–45S.
4. Comite SL, Liu JF, Balasubramanian S, et al. Treatment of HIV-associated facial lipoatrophy with Radiance FN™ (Radiesse™)//Dermatology. Online Journal 2004;10:2.
5. Jacovella PF. Use of calcium hydroxylapatite (Radiesse®) for facial augmentation. Clin Interv Aging 2008;3(1):161–74.
6. Radiesse, Merz Pharmaceuticals Electronic resource//Federal Service for Surveillance in Healthcare. URL: Available at: https://roszdravnadzor.gov.ru/services/misearch. Accessed June 16, 2021.
7. BELOTERO Soft, Merz Pharmaceuticals Electronic resource//Federal Service for Surveillance in Healthcare. URL: Available at: https://roszdravnadzor.gov.ru/services/misearch. Accessed December 12, 2022.
8. Prasetyo AD, Prager W, Rubin MG, et al. Hyaluronic acid fillers with cohesive polydensified matrix for soft-tissue augmentation and rejuvenation: a literature review. Clin Cosmet Investig Dermatol 2016;9:257–80.
9. Loghem JV, Yutskovskaya YA, Philip Werschler W. Calcium hydroxylapatite: over a decade of clinical experience. J Clin Aesthet Dermatol 2015;8(1):38–49.
10. Berlin AL, Hussain M, Goldberg DJ. Calcium hydroxylapatite filler for facial rejuvenation: a histologic and immunohistochemical analysis. Dermatol Surg 2008;34(Suppl 1):S64–7.
11. Yutskovskaya YA, Kogan EA. Improved Neocollagenesis and Skin Mechanical Properties After Injection of Diluted Calcium Hydroxylapatite in the Neck and Décolletage:A Pilot Study. J Drugs Dermatol 2017;16(1):68–74.
12. Yutskovskaya Y, Kogan E, Leshunov E. A randomized, split-face, histomorphologic study comparing a

volumetric calcium hydroxylapatite and a hyaluronic acid-based dermal filler. J Drugs Dermatol 2014; 13(9):1047–52.

13. Carruthers J, Burgess C, Day D, et al. Consensus Recommendations for Combined Aesthetic Interventions in the Face Using Botulinum Toxin, Fillers, and Energy-Based Devices. Dermatol Surg 2016;42.

14. Fabi S, Pavicic T, Braz A, et al. Combined aesthetic interventions for prevention of facial ageing, and restoration and beautification of face and body. Clin Cosmet Investig Dermatol 2017;10:423–9.

15. Suh DH, Shin MK, Lee SJ, et al. Intense focused ultrasound tightening in Asian skin: clinical and pathologic results. Dermatol Surg 2011;37(11): 1595–602.

Achieving the Attractive Asian Midface Profile with Hyaluronic Acid–Based Fillers

Wilson W.S. Ho, MBChB, FRCSEd

KEYWORDS

- Younger Asian patients for midface enhancement • Unique Asian facial anatomic features
- Improve midface projection with smaller facial appearance
- Preserve aesthetic individuality and ethnicity • Individualized treatment plan • Overfilled cheeks
- Natural result

KEY POINTS

- A larger amount of younger Asian patients seek midface enhancement because of structural deficiencies.
- The treatment goal for the Asian midface is to achieve well-projected medial cheeks and midline structures with a small and narrow-looking face.
- A customized approach is the key to creating a natural and attractive result while maintaining aesthetic individuality and Asian ethnicity.
- Volume loss compounded by tissue migration in mature patients requires combined treatment modalities for optimal results.

INTRODUCTION

Although the global hyaluronic acid (HA) -based dermal fillers market in 2020 declined by nearly 25% owing to the COVID-19 pandemic with the shutdown of aesthetic clinics, halt in supply chain, and low demand, there was a strong recovery to USD 3.89 billion in 2021, and the market is forecasted to grow to 6.93 billion USD by 2029.[1] This continuous market growth is attributed to the increasing demand for beautification and rejuvenation with increasing disposable incomes, the development of new HA products and indications with expanded treatment portfolio, the increase in awareness of HA products, and social acceptability and accessibility. The Asian market is expected to grow at the highest rate as in the past 2 decades. Moreover, the global decrease in average age for noninvasive cosmetic procedures is much earlier in Asia, and about 50% of Asian patients are aged 18 to 40 years.[2] Apart from skin quality improvement by energy-based devices, these young Asians also seek botulinum toxin and HA injections, either alone or in combination, for wrinkle removal and facial enhancement.

There are more frequent off-label uses of botulinum toxin for facial and body contouring and hence higher dosage for aesthetic indication in Asia.[3–7] Together with the regular use of intradermal botulinum toxin injections for wrinkle removal and skin quality improvement, it raised the concern of emerging trends in neurotoxin resistance and secondary nonresponse.[8,9] Nevertheless, botulinum toxin has little role in midface treatment, and HA filler is regarded as a safe, highly efficacious, and practical nonsurgical gold standard for midface enhancement. As it is common for Asians to have a wide and flat face, HA injection to midface and midline facial structures, including forehead, glabella, nose, and chin, to improve facial projection with a smaller facial appearance is a technique that every health care provider must acquire in order to practice in Asia. In mature

The Specialists: Lasers, Aesthetic and Plastic Surgery, Room 601, Prosperity Tower, 39 Queen's Road Central, Hong Kong
E-mail address: howsclinic@yahoo.com.hk

Dermatol Clin 42 (2024) 113–120
https://doi.org/10.1016/j.det.2023.06.013

Asians, it is more than addressing the lifelong mid-face structural deficiencies, but also skin atrophy, volume depletion, and tissue migration compounded by the aging process.[10] With propaganda of some filler companies and, perhaps, business consideration, it is easy to fall into the trap of trying to solve all these problems with filler and inevitably ending up with an unnatural result or even an overfilled midface. Although some of these distorted appearances will resolve spontaneously in time, others may suffer from permanent anatomic damage with persistent stigmata of an overfilled face despite medical intervention. These complications are avoidable if we respect the unique Asian midface anatomy and aesthetic ideal, conduct a thorough patient assessment with a customized treatment plan, understand the rheological properties of different HA fillers with the right choice of products, and deliver the proper aseptic and injection technique. Furthermore, adopting a multidisciplinary approach to tackle volume depletion, tissue migration, and poor skin quality is the only way to achieve a safe, reproducible, and natural result.

ASIAN MIDFACE AESTHETIC AND TREATMENT GOAL

The essential features of the midface that contribute to facial beauty and youthfulness contain malar projection and full upper cheeks with seamless transition from lower lid to cheek as well as a smooth convexity from lower eyelid down to nasolabial fold and buccal area.[11] Asians are well known to have wide bitemporal, bizygomatic, and bigonial width with short vertical facial height and flat or sometimes concave medial cheeks on the profile view.[2,12,13] When these facial features combine with depression over the temples and preauricular area, it gives rise to a typical wide, flat, and short Asian face with undereye shadow (**Fig. 1**). These structural deficiencies lead to an aesthetically undesirable masculine, tensed, aged, and hollow facial look. This unpleasant appearance will further deteriorate when the aging process takes place, in particular, with bone decay, soft tissue volume loss, and migration.

Asians usually have high, full cheekbones with retruded medial maxilla.[14] Therefore, the aim of midface rejuvenation in Asians is to project the medial cheeks without widening the malar. By projecting the medial cheeks, it will shift the light reflection points of the upper cheeks medially and create a visual impression of a small narrow-looking midface. This is a common trick that will be further magnified by removing the shadow over temporal and preauricular areas and projecting the midline facial structures. Hence, HA injection into the midface is often part of a pan-facial treatment plan with the ultimate goal of achieving an oval facial shape with increased facial height and projection. This is salient for both beautification and rejuvenation in young and mature patients, as Asians adore the youthfulness and femininity of an oval facial shape, which is gender specific and universal across all ethnicities.[14,15] With facial deflation and sagging in aging process, this youthful oval facial shape will gradually become rectangular with broken lines and angulations. Along with the loss of three-dimensionality, tissue repositioning becomes mandatory in addition to filling in order to achieve a natural and balanced result. Absorbable thread is the most popular nonsurgical option for midface lift in Asia and is sometimes the only treatment required for midface rejuvenation (**Fig. 2**). In other words, not every patient needs HA filler in rejuvenation treatment.

PATIENT ASSESSMENT

It is easy to inject but hard to obtain an attractive and balanced result while maintaining aesthetic individuality and unique ethnic characteristics. HA injection can also have severe potential complications like overfilling with permanently distorted facial appearance, tissue necrosis, and blindness. It is a medical procedure and should be regarded as being serious as any other medical treatment. A comprehensive medical history, especially history that may affect the outcome or increase the risk of complications, in particular, previous facial surgery, filler or biostimulant injection, dental caries, allergy to HA filler, and autoimmune disease. A thorough total facial assessment with the patient sitting upright in both static and in animation is crucial in arriving at a holistic treatment plan and treatment priority. Taking photographs of the whole face from different angles before injecting the patient, immediately after injection as well as in follow-up, is suggested for best practice and proper medical record.

INJECTION STRATEGY AND TECHNIQUE

Midface injection, in most circumstances, is to provide static structural support for the superficial mobile layers to glide on. Injection should be deep to the supraperiosteal level targeting the deep fat pads, namely, the lateral suborbicularis oculi fat (SOOF), medial SOOF, and deep medial cheek fat (DMCF).[16] Stiff HA gel with high elasticity and cohesivity offering strong structural support is

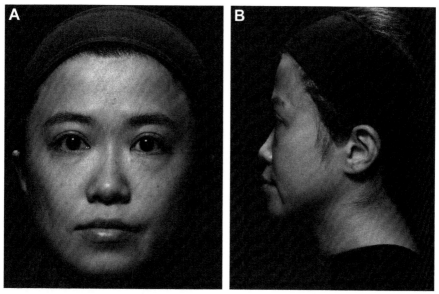

Fig. 1. (*A*) Typical morphologic features of an Asian woman illustrating the full cheekbones with flat medial cheeks and hollowness over temporal and subzygomatic regions, resulting in a wide, flat, and short face. (*B*) Profile view revealing retruded maxilla with undereye shadow and poorly projected forehead and nasal dorsum.

the product of choice especially in men and young patients. The midface is flatter and more angulated in men, and treatment should be more conservative, especially the medial cheek. A needle is preferred by most of the Asian doctors, as it is more precise and easy to control. However, a cannula is used for the fanning technique when superficial injection is required. Because treatment of

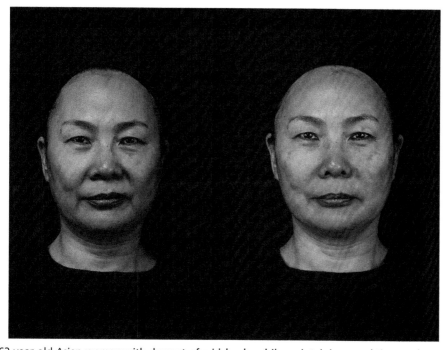

Fig. 2. A 63-year-old Asian woman with descent of midcheeks while maintaining good tissue volume. Cheek lift was done by using absorbable PDO (polydioxanone) barbed threads under local anesthesia. In addition to cheek rejuvenation, there were improvement in nasolabial folds and marionette lines, and elevation of eyebrows as a result of relaxation of the tensed orbicularis oculi muscles after getting structural support from repositioned SOOF. (*left*) Before, (*right*) immediately after, treatment.

one area will have an impact on other areas, midface injection should start from lateral to medial.[11,17,18] Treatment of the lateral cheek aiming at lateral SOOF projects and lifts the cheek with additional improvement in tear trough, nasolabial fold, jowl line, and marionette line and supports the lateral canthus.[11,18] Needle injection perpendicular to the skin all the way down to the bone will avoid trapping the HA product between the malar septum and the skin, causing the problematic malar edema. Lateral cheek injection should be very conservative in Asians, not widening the midface, as most of them have high full cheeks. The typical volume here is less than 0.15 mL per side with small boluses of 0.05 to 0.01 mL per bolus.

Medial cheek, also known as "apple cheek" in East Asia, is the most common area for filler enhancement. Injection begins from lateral canthus to a midpupillary line, targeting medial SOOF in 2 to 3 injection points with an average amount of 0.3 to 0.5 mL per side in small boluses. Stay close to the infraorbital rim just below the orbicularis retaining ligament to ensure natural youthful results and to minimize the risk of injecting the HA product into the infraorbital artery. This will also correct the palpebromalar groove, tear trough, and the V-frame deformity, which is the depression in between. Although the more HA product that is added close to the midpupillary line, the narrower the midface will be perceived, too much filler in this area will create an artificial look. Be cautious if injection is performed medial to the midpupillary line, as it is an unusual area to fill and may end up looking weird. Most young Asians with midface structural deficiencies do not need DMCF or superficial injection, and unnecessary injections will produce too much fullness in the medial cheeks. Nevertheless, DMCF injection is required in older patients with obvious soft tissue atrophy and descent of the midcheek. This is often combined with a superficial injection with soft HA gel of high cohesivity and low elasticity, which is easy to spread and resilient to repeated facial movements without causing surface irregularity or stiffness. However, midcheek tissue repositioning should come first before filling in this group of patients. In the real world, unfortunately, most of them can only afford filler, and the injector must be mindful not to overfill them by trying to solve all the aging problems with HA filler.

After taking the clinical photographs, marking and injection are done under good lighting with the patient in the supine position (**Fig. 3**). Apply an ice pack before and after the procedure over the injection area to reduce the pain and risk of bruising. Topical anesthetic cream may be used

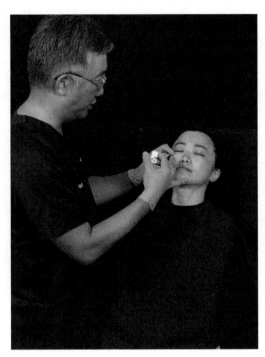

Fig. 3. Marking and injection are done under good lighting with the patient in the supine position. Apply an ice pack before and after the procedure and cleanse the injection area thoroughly with 0.05% chlorhexidine. Inject with both hands and use the noninjecting hand to guide the needle or cannula to the right tissue plane and control the HA product from spreading.

in the patient who is pain sensitive. Disinfect the injection area thoroughly with 0.05% chlorhexidine; alcohol is not preferred, as it may cause skin irritation. Inject with both hands, using the noninjecting hand to guide the needle or cannula to the right tissue plane and control the HA product from spreading. A small bolus injection is advised for safe and natural results. Inject slowly under low pressure to avoid an accidental big bolus injection and to decrease the risk of an intravascular event. Stop injection immediately if there is blanching or disproportionate pain, especially pain outside injection area, which may indicate intravascular injection. Massage gently if there is any surface irregularity and apply antibiotic cream to the needle entry point after finishing the injection. Immediate postinjection photographs should be taken routinely for best practice. It is wise to keep the patient in clinic for at least 30 minutes until the capillary refill is back to normal in case of a vascular complication, which is doubtful. Do not hesitate to inject HA if still in doubt of tissue ischemia and call for help whenever necessary.

The standard volume for midface HA injection in Asians is 1 to 2 mL in total and mostly 1 mL. In patients with severe volume depletion who need more than 2 mL, it is better to inject in separate sessions with a 2-week interval to prevent prolonged swelling, distension discomfort, and unnatural results. Maintenance can be done on a yearly basis because HA fillers nowadays can last 12 to 18 months. It is safe and effective to have other concomitant nonsurgical treatment modalities like botulinum toxin, high-energy–based devices, and thread lift without compromising the result.

POSTINJECTION CARE

Mild swelling and erythema over the injected area are common and usually subside spontaneously in 1 to 2 days. Gentle facial cleansing is allowed if needed, but no alcohol, sauna, or strenuous exercise on the day of injection, and no massage or makeup over the injected area for 24 hours. Patients should be able to go back to work immediately and are advised to come back if there is any excessive swelling, persistent pain, or mottled discoloration.

COMPLICATION MANAGEMENT

Most of the complications in midface filler injection, like swelling, erythema, and bruising, are mild and transient. However, there are more and more incidents of overfilled cheeks after repeated large-volume injections that deserve more attention. It is often driven by the desire to have drastic visible results or to aking a profit over the patient's best interests. This is alarming because repeated large-volume injections will not only produce unnatural results but also increase the risk of vascular occlusion, nodule formation, persistent swelling, product migration, and delayed inflammatory reaction. Anatomic structures can be damaged in some longstanding cases, causing permanent facial distortion. Apart from an overdose with HA fillers, overfilled cheeks may also be due to poor patient selection, improper technique by injecting the filler into incorrect tissue plane, wrong choice of product, lack of knowledge on anatomy and morphologic changes of aging, and ignoring the aesthetic ideal. Multiple attempts to dissolve the HA fillers with hyaluronidase are usually required to correct the distortion but may not be able to restore to the original look. This can be disabling and may impose enormous emotional, social, and physical stress on the patient. On the other hand, some patients will develop a distorted perception of beauty over time and pursue more filling instead of remedial treatment. That is the reason so many celebrities proudly appear on screen with overfilled cheeks.

Prevention is always better than cure, and less is more. Injecting conservatively with small boluses and addressing different aging changes with a multidisciplinary approach are the keys to preventing overfilling.

An intravascular event is uncommon in midface filler injection. However, it can still happen in experienced hands because of the distorted anatomy from previous filler injection or surgery and vascular variants. Slow and small bolus injections under low pressure with the injection needle moving continuously as though you are inside a blood vessel can reduce the risk of an intravascular event. Stop the injection if there is blanching or disproportionate pain, in particular, pain outside of the injection area. As early diagnosis and prompt hyaluronidase treatment are fundamental for uneventful recovery, hyaluronidase must be available all the time for emergency use. In a multinational survey of experienced injectors conducted by Goodman and colleagues[19] on intravascular injection with facial fillers, 86% of intravascular occlusion was resolved within 14 days, and 7% suffered moderate scarring requiring surface treatments. Minor livedo, pallor, and pain were the most frequent initial signs, but 47% of events had no pain or mild pain only. Alam and colleagues[20] found that filler injections were associated with very low risk of intravascular occlusion with either needles or cannulas and never exceeded 1 per 5000 syringes injected. However, multivariate analysis revealed that cannula had 77.1% lower odds of occlusions compared with needle injections.

CASE ILLUSTRATION
Case 1

A 55-year-old Asian woman presented with midface volume loss, V-frame deformity, and sagging (**Fig. 4**A). She had 1 mL HA injected to the midface starting from lateral to medial in 4 injection points aiming at medial SOOF. Her midface looked smaller, as the projected medial cheeks shifted the light reflection points medially. She looked rejuvenated and more refreshed with improvement in undereye shadow and nasolabial folds immediately after the injection (**Fig. 4**B).

Case 2

A 42-year-old Asian man complained of looking tired with skin laxity after rapid massive weight loss (**Fig. 5**, upper). He was treated with 400 lines of microfocused ultrasound with visualization targeted at superficial musculoaponeurotic system (SMAS) and 200 lines of synchronous ultrasound parallel beam (SUPERB) aimed at dermis; HA

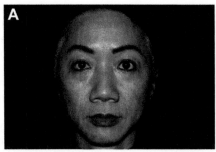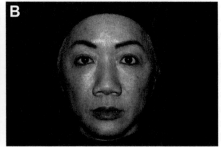

Fig. 4. (*A*) A middle-aged woman with midface descent, volume loss, and V-frame deformity. (*B*) 1 mL HA was injected to the medial cheeks starting from lateral to medial targeting the medial SOOF. The projected medial cheeks shifted the light reflection points medially, resulting in a smaller-looking midface. She looked more refreshed and rejuvenated with improvement in undereye shadow and nasolabial folds immediately after the injection.

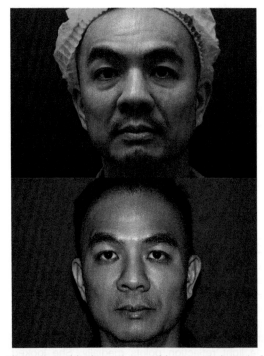

Fig. 5. A tired-looking 42-year-old man complained of facial sagging with tear troughs and prominent nasolabial folds after rapid massive weight loss. He looked much younger and masculine with better skin quality, more angulated cheeks, and well-defined jawlines after combination therapy of 400 lines of microfocused ultrasound with visualization targeted at SMAS, 200 lines of synchronous ultrasound parallel beam (SUPERB) aimed at dermis, HA injection of 2 mL to cheekbones and jawlines, 2 mL to medial cheeks, 2 mL to palpebromalar grooves and tear troughs in 2 separate sessions. (*upper*) Before, (*lower*) after, treatment. (Photo courtesy of Dr. Smith Arayaskul, MD, Bangkok, Thailand).

injection of 2 mL to the cheekbones and jawlines, 2 mL to the medial cheeks, 2 mL to the palpebromalar grooves, and tear troughs in 2 treatment sessions. Apart from improvement in skin quality, eyebags, and nasolabial folds, he looked much younger and masculine with more angulated cheeks and better defined jawlines (see **Fig. 5**, lower).

DISCUSSION

In Asia, HA fillers are most frequently used in the enhancement of the middle third of the face either as a stand-alone treatment or as part of the panfacial beautification procedure. Injecting HA fillers deep to the supraperiosteal level, aiming at deep fat pads, can provide structural support to the superficial mobile layers and modify facial muscle dynamics.[21] Although the role of filler in myomodulation is unclear, it is often to see eyebrow elevation after filler injection to SOOF or SOOF repositioning after midcheek lift by threads (see **Fig. 2**). The most likely explanation is that the orbicularis oculi muscle becomes tensed because of lack of structural support from structural deficiency, volume loss, or midcheek descent. SOOF enhancement by filler or SOOF repositioning by midcheek lift provides a stable platform and relaxes the hyperactive orbicularis oculi muscle and hence the brow elevation. This myomodulation phenomenon is also seen in other facial areas like the fading of a cobblestone appearance with the relaxation of hyperactive mentalis after filler injection to the chin. Therefore, the shift in facial muscle dynamics or rebalance of muscle activity between agonist and antagonist facial muscles may also contribute to the rejuvenation effect of filler both at rest and on animation. With that, the myomodulatory effect of filler should be taken into account first before botulinum toxin injection.

The midface is a highly mobile area. Fillers in this location need to sustain the stress of repeated compression and shearing force. Products with high elasticity, plasticity, and viscosity should be used in deep injection for structural support, and fillers with high cohesivity, low viscosity, and good tissue integration should be used in superficial mobile layers for a natural dynamic result. Inappropriate choice of fillers can result in irregularity, lumpiness, overfilling, persistent swelling, and an unnatural frozen look. Among all the possible complications of midface filler injection, sadly, overfilled cheeks have become one of the worst unwanted outcomes seen nowadays, which can cause permanent facial disfigurement. Stigmata of the distorted face also inflicts tremendous social and psychological trauma that may not response to therapeutic intervention. Perhaps, the most common reason for overfilling is poor understanding of the morphologic changes in aging. Besides volume loss from bone resorption and atrophy of deep fat compartments, descent of superficial fat pads also aggravates the hollow midface appearance in the aging process.[22] Trying to lift up the ptotic cheeks with fillers alone will inevitably end up in overfilling. Cotofana and colleagues[23] found that the transverse facial septum, a septum originated from the underside of zygomaticus major muscle forming a transversely running boundary between the buccal space and the deep midfacial fat compartments, can be the anatomic structure responsible for the overfilled midface appearance that exaggerates the facial distortion in facial movements. Knowing the anatomic characteristics and aesthetic ideal in Asians and injecting conservatively are essential in preventing overfilling. Treatment focus of midface filler injection is on medial cheeks in Asians in contrast to cheekbones in whites. Treatment endpoints should be more subtle in Asians in order to maintain discrete ethnic features and conservative cultural background. A customized multidisciplinary approach in mature patients is the key to achieving safe and natural results.

SUMMARY

A greater amount of younger Asian patients demand midface enhancement to address their structural deficiencies. Injection should be deep, targeting mainly the medial SOOF to provide structural support to orbicularis oculi muscle, improve medial cheek projection, and create a visual impression of a narrower midface by shifting the light reflection point medially. A smaller-looking midface with good projection is an essential feature of facial beauty and youthfulness, particularly in Asians. Nevertheless, it is challenging to achieve a safe and natural result. A sound knowledge of anatomy and morphologic changes in aging, a tailored treatment plan in regard to age, gender, unique Asian midface aesthetic, and cultural background, combined with proper filler selection, injection technique, and artistic sense, are the key elements to creating a youthful and attractive result.

CLINICS CARE POINTS

- The goal of midface injection in Asian patients is to project the medial cheeks and midline facial structures to create a smaller-looking face with better three-dimensionality while maintaining discrete ethnic features and aesthetic individuality.
- Injection should start from lateral to medial targeting the suborbicularis oculi fat and deep medial cheek fat if necessary.
- Conservative injections with a customized holistic treatment approach to achieve a balanced and natural result without overfilling is the goal.

DISCLOSURE

The author has no financial interests to declare in relation to the drugs, devices, and products mentioned in this article.

REFERENCES

1. Hyaluronic acid based dermal fillers market size, share & COVID-19 impact analysis, by crosslinking type, by application, by end-user, and regional forecast, 2022-2029. Fortune Business Insights Oct,2022.
2. Liew S, Wu WTL, Chan HH, et al. Consensus on changing trends, attitudes, and concepts of Asian beauty. Aesthetic Plast Surg 2016;40(2):193–201.
3. Cheng J, Hsu SH, McGee JS. Botulinum toxin injections for masseter reduction in East Asians. Dermatol Surg 2019;45(4):566–72.
4. Yu CC, Chen PK, Chen YR. Botulinum toxin A for lower facial contouring: a prospective study. Aesthetic Plast Surg 2007;31(5):445–51.
5. To EW, Ahuja AT, Ho WS, et al. A prospective study of the effect of botulinum toxin A on masseteric muscle hypertrophy with ultrasonographic and electromyographic measurement. Br J Plast Surg 2001;54(3):197–200.
6. Zhou RR, Wu HL, Zhang XD, et al. Efficacy and safety of botulinum toxin type A injection in patients

with bilateral trapezius hypertrophy. Aesthetic Plast Surg 2018;42(6):1664–71.

7. Cheng J, Chung HJ, Friedland M, et al. Botulinum toxin injections for leg contouring in East Asians. Dermatol Surg 2020;46(Suppl 1):S62–70.

8. Park JY, Cho SI, Hur K, et al. Intradermal microdroplet injection of diluted incobotulinumtoxin-A for sebum control, face lifting, and pore size improvement. J Drugs Dermatol 2021;20(1):49–54.

9. Ho WWS, Albrecht P, Calderon PE, et al. Emerging trends in botulinum neurotoxin A resistance: an international multidisciplinary review and consensus. Plast Reconstr Surg Glob Open 2022;10(6):e4407.

10. Ho WWS. Facial beautification and rejuvenation with injectables: my preferred approach. Clin Plast Surg 2023;50(1):11–7.

11. de Maio M, DeBoulle K, Braz A, et al. Facial assessment and injection guide for botulinum toxin and injectable hyaluronic acid fillers: focus on the midface. Plast Reconstr Surg 2017;140(4):540e–50e.

12. Le TT, Farkas LG, Ngim RC, et al. Proportionality in Asian and North American Caucasian faces using neoclassical facial canons as criteria. Aesthetic Plast Surg 2002;26(1):64–9.

13. Gu Y, McNamara JA Jr, Sigler LM, et al. Comparison of craniofacial characteristics of typical Chinese and Caucasian young adults. Eur J Orthod 2011;33(2):205–11.

14. Wu WTL, Liew S, Chan HH, et al. Consensus on current injectable treatment strategies in the Asian face. Aesthetic Plast Surg 2016;40(2):202–14.

15. Goodman GJ. The oval female facial shape – a study in beauty. Dermatol Surg 2015;41(12):1375–83.

16. Trévidic P, Weinkle JKS, Wu R, et al. Injection guidelines for treating midface volume deficiency with hyaluronic acid fillers: the ATP approach (anatomy, techniques, products). Aesthet Surg J 2022;42(8):920–34.

17. Shamban A, Clague MD, von Grote E, et al. A novel and more aesthetic injection pattern for malar cheek volume restoration. Aesthetic Plast Surg 2018;42(1):197–200.

18. Van Loghem J, Sattler S, Casabona G, et al. Consensus on the use of hyaluronic acid fillers from the cohesive polydensified matrix range: best practice in specific facial indications. Clin Cosmet Investig Dermatol 2021;14:1175–99.

19. Goodman GJ, Roberts S, Callan P. Experience and management of intravascular injection with facial fillers: results of a multinational survey of experienced injectors. Aesthetic Plastic Surg 2016;40(4):549–55.

20. Alam M, Kakar R, Dover JS, et al. Rates of vascular occlusion associated with using needles vs cannulas for filler injection. JAMA Dermatol 2021;157(2):174–80.

21. de Maio M. Myomodulation with injectables fillers: an innovative approach to addressing facial muscle movement. Aesthetic Plastic Surg 2018;42(3):798–814.

22. Farkas JP, Pessa JE, Hubbard B, et al. The science and theory behind facial aging. Plast Reconstr Surg Glob Open 2013;1(1):E8–15.

23. Cotofana S, Gotkin RH, Frank K, et al. Anatomy behind the facial overfilled syndrome: the transverse facial septum. Dermatol Surg 2020;46(8):e16–22.

Facial Overfilled Syndrome

Tingsong Lim, MD

KEYWORDS

- Facial overfilled syndrome • Complications • Distortion • Filler overused • Facial topography
- Unnatural outcome • Fillers • Injectables

KEY POINTS

- Facial overfilled syndrome is an underdiagnosed aesthetic complication due to multiple incorrect placements of fillers.
- Incorrectly placed dermal fillers, poor selection of filler products, overzealous attempts by the injectors, and overly enthusiastic clients who "chase the lines" are the common causes of this phenomenon.
- We have experienced massive advancements in aesthetic medicine, in terms of not only technology but also our approach in refining and restoring beauty and youth in a person.
- Facial overfilled syndrome is a phenomenon that is becoming more common due to accumulative overuse of hyaluronic acid (HA) or non-HA fillers on the face.

FACIAL OVERFILLED SYNDROME

For the past decade or so, we have experienced massive advancements in aesthetic medicine, in terms of not only technology but also our approach in refining and restoring beauty and youth in a person. In that process, we have stumbled on some unexpected and sometimes unfavourable outcomes during our quests in perfecting our artistry in this field.

One of the most common but hardly talked about complications is facial overfilled syndrome (FOS). FOS is a phenomenon that is becoming more common due to accumulative overuse of hyaluronic acid (HA) or non-HA fillers on the face. It can be seen among those who had volume overload in the midface, forehead, chin, and nose. Incorrectly placed dermal fillers, poor selection of filler products, overzealous attempts by the injectors, and overly enthusiastic clients who "chase the lines" are the common causes of this phenomenon. FOS does not happen overnight, but it is a consequence of progressive volume addition to the face after a series of high-dose filler injections.

Facial fillers are injectable substances that are used to add volume to the face, enhance facial features, and reduce the appearance of wrinkles and fine lines. These fillers are commonly used to plump up the lips, cheeks, and undereye areas. The most used fillers are HA, collagen, and poly-L-lactic acid. Although these fillers are generally considered safe, they can cause complications if used excessively. FOS occurs when a person receives too many fillers or when the fillers are injected in the wrong areas of the face; this results in an unnatural, distorted appearance that can be difficult to correct. FOS can occur in both men and women of all ages, but it is more commonly seen in older individuals who have received numerous injections over time.

Many of those who have FOS lose their original facial topography and may or may not be aware of their condition. In fact, facial distortion due to the overfilled syndrome normally becomes more apparent as one ages, exaggerated by tissue sagging. In the early phases, FOS can be picked up during facial expressions and movements. FOS is more commonly "produced" by practitioners depending solely on a single modality of treatment.

This syndrome is underdiagnosed, and many practitioners are not aware of such conditions. In fact, studies have shown that visual adaptation happens when one is frequently exposed to extreme volume in the face, that one would regard overfilled faces as normal.[1] Having the awareness

Clique Clinic, 4, Jalan 19/36, Petaling Jaya, Selangor 46300, Malaysia
E-mail address: drlim@cliqueclinic.com

Dermatol Clin 42 (2024) 121–128
https://doi.org/10.1016/j.det.2023.06.007

derm.theclinics.com

of the overfilled syndrome is crucial among aesthetic practitioners to prevent it from happening. Once a face is overfilled and the structure is distorted, diminishing the volume with hyaluronidase will help to minimize the distortion but will not necessarily restore the face to its natural look. Therefore, it is very important for the medical aesthetic community to bring up the awareness of overfilled syndrome and prevent this from happening.

CAUSES OF FACIAL OVERFILLED SYNDROME

There are several factors that contribute to the development of FOS. One of the primary causes is the lack of awareness in the aesthetics industry. Many people are performing injectable treatments without proper training or certification and have been doing the treatment based on the theory that facial aging is due to volume loss. Based on that logic, it only makes sense to inject as many fillers as possible into the face to "combat" the signs of aging. However, placing large volume of fillers into the face would also increase the weight of the soft tissues of the face and expedite aging signs. Many would think that it is safe to have big amounts of fillers placed into the soft tissues, as most HA fillers will disappear with time. We have seen many of the overfilled faces continue to carry the fillers with them despite having no new fillers added to them for many years, making many question if the HA fillers actually go away with time.

FOS is also caused by incorrect assessment, injection plane and techniques, choice of products, and volume administered. As we age, the face undergoes dynamic, cumulative transformations of the tissue structure due to the combined effects of bone resorption, weakening of the anchoring complex, facial muscle behavior changes, and soft tissue mispositioning. Superficial subcutaneous fat of the face does not deplete in volume but in fact increases in volume with aging.[2] Deep subcutaneous facial fat decreases in volume, but only on the upper one-third of the fat pads, but the lower two-thirds of the fat pad is seen to increase in volume with aging. This increase can be mostly attributed to fat pad malpositioning rather than true volume loss.

Most of these observations can be explained by a weakening of the anchoring complex: a complex structure that tethers soft tissues to facial bones. Connecting to the periosteum are the retaining ligaments and the cobweb-like areolar structures. These strong connective tissues pass through the muscles, then spread out as fiber septae, holding the fat tissues between the skin and the superficial musculo-aponeurosis system just above the muscles. This system nails the soft tissues firmly to the bone, but as it weakens with aging, we start to appreciate sagging and soft tissue mispositioning, translating into prominent eye bags, tear troughs, nasojugal lines, nasolabial folds, and jowls.[3–5]

Therefore, placing fillers into areas of the face that already have mispositioned soft tissues generally would not yield a long-standing result. Practitioners lacking such awareness will be pressured to use more fillers to create more drastic changes that would only speed up aging and cause FOS. Therefore, FOS is normally seen done by practitioners who believed in creating drastic results or conform to unrealistic beauty standards. Social media and the entertainment industry often promote a certain image of beauty that is unattainable for most people; this has led to an increased demand for cosmetic treatments, including fillers, which can result in excessive use.

FOS is frequently seen among patients of physicians who rely solely on filler treatments for lifting purposes; this highlights a prioritization of profit over artistry or lack of comprehension of the pathophysiology of aging. Although producing drastic outcomes may be desired or even requested, it is best avoided due to the risks to safety and potential for permanently distorting the patient's natural facial structure and contours.

SYMPTOMS OF FACIAL OVERFILLED SYNDROME

The primary symptom of FOS is an unnatural appearance of the face, which can include overly plumped lips, cheeks, and undereye areas. The face may also seem lumpy or asymmetrical, with some areas appearing larger than others. In severe cases, the face may become distorted, making it difficult for the individual to recognize themselves in the mirror (**Figs. 1** and **2**).

DIAGNOSIS OF FACIAL OVERFILLED SYNDROME

The diagnosis of FOS is primarily based on a physical examination of the face. A trained aesthetician or plastic surgeon can usually identify the syndrome by looking at the individual's face and assessing the distribution of the fillers. In some cases, imaging tests such as ultrasound, MRI, or computed tomography scans may be used to evaluate the distribution of the fillers and determine the best course of treatment.

Patient displays one or more of the following features[6]:

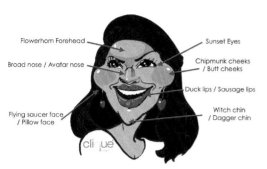

Fig. 1. The common signs of facial overfilled syndrome in a female patient.

- Loss of normal topography of the infraorbital area
- Very heavy lower midface
- Disproportionate zygomatic arch causing relatively oversunken temple
- "Setting-sun eyes" phenomenon
- Broadened nose
- Overprotruding forehead
- Pointy chin
- Sausage-like lips
- Drooping mouth corners (**Fig. 3**)

TREATMENT OPTIONS FOR FACIAL OVERFILLED SYNDROME

The treatment of FOS depends on the severity and the individual's goals. In mild cases, the fillers may gradually migrate over time, and the individual may choose to avoid further injections and continue with skin tightening procedures to prevent sagging. In more severe cases, the fillers may need to be removed. This procedure involves injecting hyaluronidase into the areas where the fillers were placed or surgical removal. The procedure is followed by aggressive skin tightening efforts to avoid sagging and skin laxity issues. In cases where the fillers have caused significant damage to the facial tissue, additional treatments such as skin resurfacing or laser therapy may be

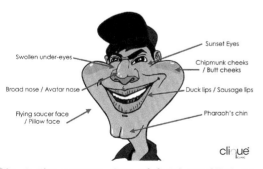

Fig. 2. The common signs of facial overfilled syndrome in a male patient.

necessary to improve the appearance of the skin (**Figs. 4** and **5**).

PREVENTION OF FACIAL OVERFILLED SYNDROME

The best way to prevent FOS is to understand the anatomy of the face and have a good grasp of the knowledge of the fillers being used. Also, trained eyes sensitive to the natural contouring or topography of the face is very important. Avoiding large boluses while injecting and working on minimal effective dosage when doing filler injection help to prevent overfilling from happening. It is also important to create widespread awareness of the possibility of such adverse effects. Overfilled syndrome could lead to an aesthetically unpleasing appearance that may worsen psychological distress and irreversibly damage tissue. Injectors must be able to immediately recognize when an overfilled condition is present and provide treatments to address it.

Normally, a true overfilled syndrome is easy to identify, as the topography of the face is overtly distorted. However, identification of a borderline overfilled syndrome is less straight forward. Simple exercises can be used to identify such overfilled conditions; palpation of the area suspected of being overfilled could be performed with both the thumb and index finger to assess the fluidity of the substance beneath the skin. The medial infraorbital area is the area most easily identified, as it is generally the thinnest-skinned area of the face, with minimal fat. By compressing the structures, a soft, fluidlike consistency, which seems translucent in light, generally confirms the diagnosis. In this study, still photos were captured but overfilled areas are most noticeable during muscle animation when filler accumulates in discrete and visible lumps beneath moving muscles. Practical management of overfilled syndrome requires the direct injection of hyaluronidase with lidocaine into the areas suspected to contain excessive fillers. It is important for the physician to identify the layers in which the fillers could have been deposited. However, it is often very difficult to detect the clear borders of filler locations.

CORRECTION OF OVERFILLED SYNDROME

Overfilled areas or lumps are identified and to be injected with 1500 IU of hyaluronidase in 5 mL of lidocaine using 30 G needles. It is imperative that this injection punctures the filler lumps and the needle penetrates the biofilm or capsule surrounding the filler mass. In most cases, a few sessions of

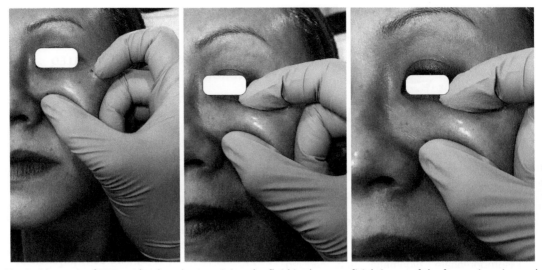

Fig. 3. Diagnosis of FOS can be done by examining the fluid in the superficial tissues of the face or imaging such as ultrasound, computed tomography (CT) scans and MRI.

hyaluronidase are needed to have prominent correction. The longer the fillers have been in the tissues, the harder it is to be dissolved. Also, the more cross-linking an injected filler has, the more hyaluronidase is needed to breakdown the residual product.

Injections are performed at multiple depths and angles in the hope of penetrating multiple biofilms or capsulations to allow hyaluronidase to work. Multiple sessions of hyaluronidase treatments may be needed to achieve significant volume changes. The use of hyaluronidase may be less effective if filler implants have been present for a longer time, performed in multiple sessions, or have migrated extensively. In medicine, prevention is always better than cure and it is important to create awareness among practitioners on the severity of the overfilled syndrome. Many

physicians do not consider overfilling to be problematic, as they assume that this will resolve naturally after several years. As the overfilled structure is generally unable to withstand gravity and aging, the distortion worsens with age, eventually leading to an unnatural looking face (**Figs. 6–9**).

THIS IS JUST THE BEGINNING

More research with histological studies on filler longevity and their impact on the deep fat layers is required. It is also important to identify the volumetric changes that occur with aging and to correct this accordingly. Most midface deflation was believed to be due to suborbicularis oculi fat (SOOF) volume depletion.[7–10] A normal person has 2 to 3 mL of SOOF volume at adulthood. In the author's opinion, should depletion of fat occur

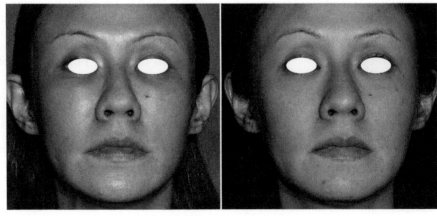

Fig. 4. Managing FOS with hyaluronidase injections.

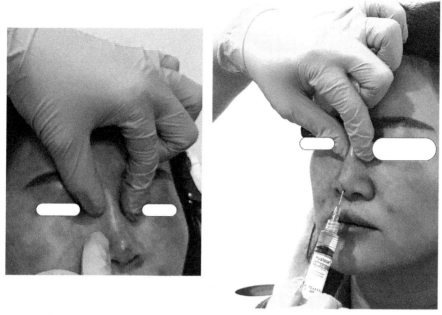

Fig. 5. Correction of overfilled nose with hyaluronidase.

at a rate of 1% to 2% per year, a maintenance dose of 0.02 to 0.06 mL of fillers would be needed per year. To correct 10 years of volume loss, an estimation of not more than 0.2 to 0.6 mL of filler should be deposited only once and a maintenance dose subsequently continued.

It would also be interesting to determine the distribution of fillers after placement underneath the skin. With larger boluses, it is quite possible that fillers are more prone to migrate or be "squeezed" to other areas, hence losing their projection and causing a wider spread of fillers to unfavorable areas. Conducting studies that compare the migration rates of fillers of different volumes and of different rheology will help physicians understand the volumetric limits underneath the skin.

It is hard to be certain that fillers are placed correctly in the intended area of fat, bone, or soft tissue loss. Similarly, if the amount of fat and bone loss or other factors are taken into consideration, simply adding 4 to 5 mL of filler in the cheek area can produce an exaggerated, overfilled appearance. Practical management of overfilled syndrome requires the direct injection of hyaluronidase with lidocaine into the areas suspected to contain excessive fillers.

Hyaluronidase exists predominantly in the skin, but fillers are generally injected subcutaneously or deeper, thus precluding filler removal unless treated with surgical excision or an immune-based disintegrative reaction or filler migration away from the point of injection. Occasionally after

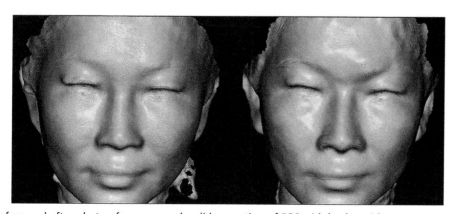

Fig. 6. Before and after photo of a woman who did correction of FOS with hyaluronidase.

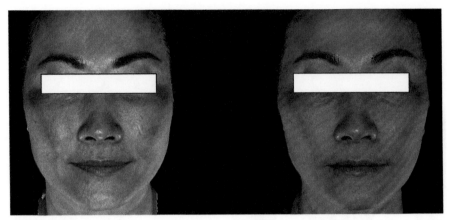

Fig. 7. (Front view) Before and after photo of a woman who did correction of FOS with hyaluronidase.

treatment, when patients view their treated area, they notice a flattening of the area. This flattening does not result from filler disintegration but is due to filler spread or migration away from the intended target site. Overfilled syndrome does not necessarily occur after a single session or after the use of excessive filler volumes. Of greater importance is the fact that it now more commonly occurs after several years of filler use and the unintended accumulation of filler in a specific site. Although some fillers are thought to be biodegradable, this has not been proved. It is plausible that filler particles continue to exist for several years and may migrate to or integrate with unintended tissue layers.

Injection of large boluses creates more tension within the treated tissues, prompting an immune response that creates a biofilm or fibrous "cage" around the foreign body. To remove these bodies, it is necessary to inject hyaluronidase directly into the masses. Many patients claim to not have received any filler injections in the prior 5 to 6 years and yet still seem overfilled or filled; this has prompted the question of whether biodegradable fillers do completely disintegrate and whether the mass leading to the overfilled appearance is composed of collagen fibers. In the latter instance, treatment with hyaluronidase immediately eliminates the mass, indicating that the mass was indeed created by fillers. It is essential to note that during hyaluronidase treatment, mere flooding of the filler-filled area does not eliminate the mass, as the hyaluronidase is unable to penetrate the biofilm cage surrounding the filler mass. To remove such lumps, multiple needle punctures must be delivered to the site to ensure that one or more biofilm-caged filler masses have been directly injected with hyaluronidase. After this, removal of the mass is effortless. Once a face is overfilled and the native tissue structure becomes distorted, diminishing the supplementary volume with hyaluronidase will help minimize distortions but may not necessarily restore a natural appearance. Therefore, it is very important for the medical

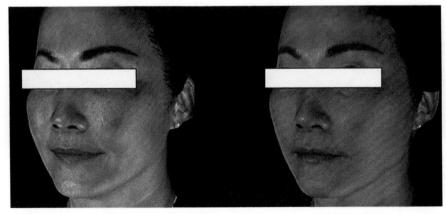

Fig. 8. (Left view) Before and after photo of a woman who did correction of FOS with hyaluronidase.

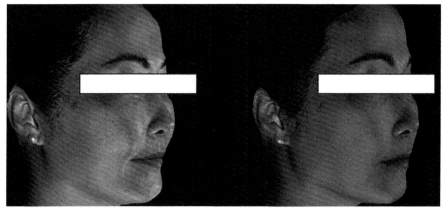

Fig. 9. (Right view) Before and after photo of a woman who did correction of FOS with hyaluronidase.

aesthetic community to increase patient awareness of overfilled syndrome to prevent this from occurring.

Aesthetic practitioners must try to avoid overfilling and learn to apply caution to their filler selection, volume used, and chosen location.[11] By ensuring that practitioners are not deliberately causing harm by overfilling, the quality of aesthetic medical outcomes also improves. One way of facilitating this process is to understand how the 5 key tissues in the face, namely the skin, fat, anchoring complex, muscles, and bones, contribute to aging. It is vital to target aging in all 5 layers by combining different modalities and acknowledge that this strategy has now come of age—combination treatment approaches are no longer simply a trend but have evolved to become a necessity.

SUMMARY

Replenishing volume to attain a more youthful appearance yields excellent results, enabling the deflating face to regain volume and firmness. This phenomenon of mild-to-severe facial distortion induced by incorrectly used dermal fillers is especially apparent among Asian patients who have smaller bone structures within the mongoloid skull. Having an awareness of the overfilled syndrome is instrumental among aesthetic practitioners in preventing the creation of distorted, unnatural, and aesthetically unappealing faces. The cause of overfilling is multifactorial. Incorrect assessment due to lack of experience or training, incorrect filler placement in fat compartments (such as the superficial fat pads or medial infraorbital areas), poor selection of product, and problematic injection techniques can all lead to the overfilled syndrome. Often, an

incorrect volume of filler is delivered due to physician overzealousness and desire to produce a "wow" effect but can distort the facial structure. Repeatedly placing fillers in the same tissue compartment over multiple treatment sessions is generally the cause.

CLINICS CARE POINTS

- Always use small amount of fillers (preferably less than 0.1ml per area)
- Avoid doing bolus injection, let it be sharp needlee or cannula
- microdroplets and dispersing the HA fillers at multiple layers and precise innoculation is the best way to deliver fillers
- Fillers do stay in the soft tissue of the face for a long time. Placing wrong type of fillers at the wrong place would lead to filler migration and later lead to long term complications.

DISCLOSURE

There are no commercial or financial conflicts of interest for this authorship. No funding was involved.

REFERENCES

1. Goldie K, Cumming D, Voropai D, et al. Aesthetic delusions: an investigation into the role of rapid visual adaptation in aesthetic practice. Clinical, cosmetic and investigational dermatology 2021:14 Kahn DM, Shaw RB Jr (2008) aging of the bony

orbit: a three- dimensional computed tomographic study. Aesthetic Surg J 2021;28:258–64.

2. Gosain AK1, Klein MH, Sudhakar PV, et al. A volumetric analysis of soft-tissue changes in the aging midface using high-resolution MRI: implications for facial rejuvenation. Plast Reconstr Surg 2005;115(4):1143–52 [discussion: 1153-5].

3. Rohrich RJ, Pessa JE. The retaining system of the face: histologic evaluation of the septal boundaries of the subcutaneous fat compartments. Plast Reconstr Surg 2008;121(5):1804–9.

4. Yang NZ, Wang ZJ, Wang B, et al. [Anatomic study of malar fat pad and aging analysis]. Zhonghua Zheng Xing Wai Ke Za Zhi. 2012;28(3):212-217. Chinese.

5. Buchanan DR. Wulc AE Contemporary thoughts on lower eyelid/midface aging. Clin Plast Surg 2015; 42(1):1–15.

6. Lim TS. Facial overfilled syndrome complications of inappropriate filler delivery. PRIME J 2018;6(1).

7. Hwang SH, Hwang K, Jin S, et al. Location and nature of retro-orbicularis oculus fat and suborbicularis oculi fat. J Craniofac Surg 2007;18(2):387–90.

8. Rohrich RJ, Arbique GM, Wong C, et al. The anatomy of suborbicularis fat: implications for periorbital rejuvenation. Plast Reconstr Surg 2009;124(3):946–51.

9. Matthias G, Stöhring C, Buder T, et al. Aging changes of the midfacial fat compartments: a computed tomographic study. Plast Reconstr Surg 2012;129(1):263–73.

10. Rohrich R, Pessa JE, Ristow B. The youthful cheek and the deep medial fat compartment. Plast Reconstr Surg 2008;21(121):2107–12.

11. Lim T, Frank K, Hadjab B. Target-specific sandwich technique: facial rejuvenation leveraging CPM technology. J Cosmet Dermatol 2022;21(1):207–19.

Cellulite
An Update on Pathogenesis and Management

Samar Khalil, MD[a],*, Hassan I. Galadari, MD[b]

KEYWORDS

- Cellulite • Fat • Subcision • Radiofrequency • Radiesse • Sculptra

KEY POINTS

- Cellulite is a common condition affecting most of the postpubertal women.
- Risk factors include a genetic predisposition, female gender, age, higher amounts of subcutaneous fat, Caucasian race, a sedentary lifestyle, and pregnancy.
- Different pathophysiologic mechanisms have been proposed including structural, hormonal, vascular, and inflammatory.
- Treatment remains a challenge, and combination therapy is often recommended for optimal results.

INTRODUCTION

Cellulite—also known as gynoid lipodystrophy, liposclerosis, or dermatofibrosclerosis—is a common skin condition affecting around 85% to 98% of postpubertal women. It is characterized by dimpling of the skin, leading to an "orange peel" appearance. It is most commonly seen on the thighs and buttocks.[1,2]

Risk factors include a genetic predisposition, female gender, age, Caucasian race, a sedentary lifestyle, and pregnancy. Obesity may worsen the condition but cellulite also occurs in lean women.[2,3] Despite many advances in therapeutic options, management remains a challenge because most treatments have unpredictable efficacy and durability of results.

Many women with cellulite experience emotional distress that can affect self-esteem and quality of life. In a study by Hexsel and colleagues, half of the study participants reported having received an embarrassing comment related to their cellulite and 78.3% felt compelled to seek treatment.[4]

ANATOMY AND CAUSE

Cellulite can be broken down into 3 main structural components (**Fig. 1**):

1. Clusters of adipocytes separated by bands of connective tissue;
2. Bands of connective tissue called septae, which connect the muscle to the lower aspect of the dermis at a nonflexible length; and
3. The overlying skin.[5]

It is believed that the depressed areas of cellulite result from the presence of thick fibrous septae, whereas the raised areas result from fat herniation into the weakened overlying skin.[6]

The cause of cellulite is still unclear but it is definitely multifactorial. Different pathophysiologic mechanisms have been proposed including structural, hormonal, vascular, and inflammatory.

[a] Skin & Scalpel clinic, Sin el Fil, Lebanon; [b] College of Medicine and Health Sciences, United Arab Emirates University, Al Ain, United Arab Emirates
* Corresponding author. Skin & scalpel clinic, Qubic Business Center, 10th floor, Horsh Tabet, Sin el Fil, Lebanon
E-mail address: dr.samar.khalil.00@gmail.com

Dermatol Clin 42 (2024) 129–137
https://doi.org/10.1016/j.det.2023.06.008
0733-8635/24/© 2023 Elsevier Inc. All rights reserved.

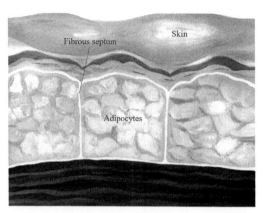

Fig. 1. The topographic alterations in cellulite are believed to be the result of herniation of fat lobules into the weakened overlying skin (raised areas) and thickening of the fibrous septae surrounding these fat lobules (dimples).

Structural

Nürnberger and Müller were the first to propose that the topographic alterations in cellulite are caused by fat herniation into a weakened dermis. The high prevalence of cellulite in women may be related to gender-specific anatomic differences. Men have obliquely oriented, criss-crossing connective tissue fibers, whereas women have perpendicularly arranged, less dense fibers. The female anatomy provides less stability, thereby accounting for the higher prevalence of cellulite in women.[7]

In a study involving 20 fresh cadavers from 10 male and 10 female Caucasian body donors, men had a greater number of subdermal fat lobules and septal connections between the superficial fascia and dermis. Furthermore, the force needed to cause septal breakage in male body donors was significantly greater than in female body donors. The mean dermal thickness was not significantly different between sexes but it decreased with increased age.[8]

In a study by Querleux and colleagues, women with cellulite had thickened adipose layers compared with men or women without cellulite.[9] Mirrashed and colleagues used MRI to demonstrate that the extent of fat protrusion into the dermis is significantly higher in women with a high cellulite grade compared with men or in women with lower cellulite grades.[10] However, Pierard and colleagues did not find a correlation between the extent of fat protrusion and the clinical severity of cellulite. They proposed that the fibrous bands separating the subcutis might represent a reactive process to sustained pressure caused by fat accumulation. Dimpling occurs when this reactive process is overcome by fat

accumulation. Therefore, bulging of fat lobules represents a secondary event.[11]

Hexsel and colleagues showed that buttock areas with cellulite depressions have significantly more fibrous septae, and these septae are thicker compared with areas without cellulite. However, the thickness of these fibrous bands did not correlate with the clinical severity of cellulite. There were no statistically significant differences in the thickness of the adipose tissue.[12]

Vascular

Curri and Bombardelli proposed that decreased blood and lymphatic flow in the subcutaneous adipose tissues could promote neovascularization and thickening of the fibrous septae.[13] In a study by Lotti and colleagues, cellulite skin had increased concentrations of glycosaminoglycans (GAGs). Terminal arterioles and dermal capillaries also had abundant deposits of granular material and scattered areas of duplicated basement membrane.[14]

The increased capillary pressure leads to increased vascular permeability and fluid retention. GAGs also raise the interstitial pressure, attracting further water. Edema eventually leads to vascular compression, decreased venous return, and tissue hypoxia. All these changes result in fibrogenesis and thickening of the interlobular septae. Furthermore, the lipolytic resistance triggered by tissue hypoxia coupled with the lipogenesis triggered by estrogen and a high carbohydrate intake causes the fat globules to become more hypertrophied and nodular.[1]

The findings of increased water retention in cellulite skin have not been replicated in other studies. In a study by Querleux and colleagues, magnetic resonance spectroscopy did not show increased water content in the adipose tissue of women with cellulite.[9] A study by Rosenbaum and colleagues showed no significant differences in subcutaneous adipose tissue morphology, lipolytic responsiveness, or regional blood flow between affected and unaffected sites.[15]

Inflammatory

Because of the tenderness on compression reported by some patients with cellulite, some investigators have suggested that inflammation is a contributor to the development of cellulite. Obesity is associated with an inflammatory response in adipose tissues characterized by the recruitment of M1 macrophages, Th1 cells, and mast cells. This local response leads to the production of proinflammatory cytokines such as tumor necrosis factor alpha and interleukin-6 and may result in endothelial damage. These cytokines have also been associated with insulin resistance and an increased risk of cardiovascular events. Some investigators have therefore suggested that cellulite is not only a cosmetic concern and may be associated with systemic diseases.[16]

Hypoxia inducible factor 1 (HIF-1) is a transcriptional activator protein made up of 2 subunits (α and β). The α subunit (HIF1A) is directly regulated by oxygen tension. HIF-1 is responsible for regulating a variety of target genes including those involved in angiogenesis, matrix metabolism, apoptosis, and glycolysis. In early stages of adipose tissue expansion, hypoxia occurs because of the lack of an adequate vascular network, and HIF1A is upregulated. High HIF1A expression initiates adipose tissue fibrosis and promotes local inflammation.[17] A genetic variant of the HIF1A gene was associated with a reduced risk for cellulite. This polymorphism leads to a reduced activity of the subunit.[18,19]

In biopsy specimens, Kligman detected the presence of a chronic inflammatory response in the fibrous septae and proposed that this response results in adipolysis and dermal atrophy.[20] Other investigators, however, found no evidence of inflammation.[7,21]

Hormonal

The anatomic landmarks predisposing to cellulite may be hormonally driven. In fact, the early signs of cellulite appear during puberty, and the condition may worsen during pregnancy, in women using birth control pills, or postmenopausal women on hormone replacement therapy. Estrogen promotes lipogenesis (through stimulation of lipoprotein lipase) and impedes lipolysis. Cellulite is uncommon in men but occurs more frequently in conditions resulting in androgen deficiency, requiring antiandrogen therapy such as Klinefelter syndrome, requiring estrogen therapy such as prostate cancer, hypogonadism, or postcastration.[1,2,22,23]

GRADING AND ASSESSMENT

Physical examination should be done with the patient standing. To accentuate skin dimpling, the patient can contract the muscles in the area or the pinch test can be done, that is, pinching the area of interest between the thumb and index finger. Overhead or tangential lighting is recommended for a better visualization of the surface topography.[5]

Nürnberger and Müller proposed the first clinical grading scale for cellulite made up of 3 grades[7] (Table 1).

Table 1 Nürnberger–Müller scale for cellulite	
Grade	**Clinical Appearance**
I	Skin is smooth at rest but the pinch test is positive.
II	Skin is smooth while the patient is lying but shows an orange peel or mattress appearance on standing.
III	Grade II cellulite plus raised and depressed areas and nodules while the patient is lying or standing.

Adapted from Nurnberger F, Muller G. So-called cellulite: an invented disease. J Dermatol Surg Oncol. 1978;4(3):221-229.

Hexsel and colleagues proposed the first validated photonumeric cellulite severity scale (CSS) based on 5 key morphologic features of cellulite[24]:

1. Number of depressions
2. Depth of depressions
3. Morphologic appearance of skin surface alterations
4. Extent of skin laxity, flaccidity, or sagging
5. Nürnberger–Müller classification grade. The severity of each item is graded from 0 to 3, leading to overall grades of mild (1–5), moderate (6–10), and severe (11–15).

Cellulite dimples—at rest and cellulite dimples—dynamic scales were developed more recently by Hexsel and colleagues for a better and faster assessment of treatment outcomes. The scales quantify the severity of cellulite dimples in both static (at rest) and dynamic states.[25]

Other cellulite grading scales include Curri scale, DiBernardo Scoring System, Clinician Reported and Patient Reported Photonumeric Cellulite Severity Scales, and Investigator and Subjective Global Aesthetic Improvement Scales.[26]

Several imaging modalities have been used to evaluate cellulite severity including 2-dimensional (2D) or 3D digital photography, ultrasonography, and MRI. Measurements of skin biomechanics (eg, elasticity) have also been used in some studies. Photographic assessment of cellulite is currently the only validated modality, and thus the Food and Drug Administration (FDA) has recommended that assessments of treatment efficacy should use photonumeric scales.[26]

TREATMENT

In recent years, a better understanding of cellulite has led to the development of new treatments that target the different etiologic factors involved in the pathogenesis of the condition. Unfortunately, there is little scientific evidence to support the efficacy of these treatments. Physicians should make their patients aware of the unpredictable efficacy of treatment and the potential for only short-term improvement despite numerous treatment sessions. Oftentimes, combining different therapeutic modalities is advised to achieve more noticeable and sustained results.[1]

Attenuation of Aggravating Factors

A well-balanced diet is often recommended for cellulite. The ideal diet varies between one patient and another but, in general, excessive intake of fats, carbohydrates, and salt should be avoided.[27]

Regular exercise is also recommended to increase blood flow to adipose tissues, promote lipolysis and weight loss, and increase muscle strength. It is not clear which type of exercise training (endurance, resistance, or combined training) is optimal to achieve the best outcomes.[28]

It must be noted that cellulite occurs in both obese and lean women, and there is very little evidence supporting the positive impact of weight loss on cellulite. In a study by Smalls and colleagues, weight loss improved the appearance of cellulite in most of the patients but worsened it in others. Improvement was associated with significant reductions in weight and percentage of thigh fat, significantly higher starting body mass index, and significantly greater initial cellulite severity. Worsening was associated with a significantly smaller starting body mass index, smaller reductions in weight accompanied by no change in percentage of thigh fat, and significant increases in tissue compliance.[29]

Topical Treatments

The main active ingredients used in topical preparations are xanthines (caffeine, aminophylline, and theophylline), retinoids, and various botanic extracts. Possible mechanisms of action include stimulation of lipolysis, improved microcirculation, reduced inflammation, and increased neocollagenesis. Xanthines are believed to work through inhibiting phosphodiesterase and increasing adenosine monophosphate levels in adipocytes, thus stimulating lipolysis. A systematic review of 21 studies assessing the efficacy of topical products in cellulite reduction concluded that they have a moderate efficacy in thigh circumference reduction. However, most of these studies had methodological or reporting flaws. Larger randomized controlled trials are required to assess the efficacy of topical formulations in the treatment of cellulite.[30]

Massage

LPG endermologie is a US FDA-approved treatment of cellulite. It was designed by a French engineer, Louis Paul Guitay, and bears his initials. The device exerts positive pressure via 2 rollers and negative pressure via an aspiration system. This technique likely works by promoting lymphatic drainage and redistributing extracellular fluid. Evidence supporting its efficacy remains scant. In an observational study, 69% of participants were highly satisfied after at least 15 sessions of endermologie performed twice weekly.[31] In another study, only 5 of 33 subjects had a reduction in cellulite grade after 15 sessions.[32] In both studies, there is no mention of the durability of results. From clinical experience, improvement is short-lived and maintenance therapy is advised.

Extracorporeal Shock Wave Therapy

Extracorporeal shock wave therapy (ESWT) uses electrical energy to create mechanical disruption of tissues, resulting in a healing response, collagen remodeling, neovascularization, and improved lymphatic drainage. Furthermore, shockwaves weaken the fibrous septae and smoothen the afflicted skin. Typically, 1 or 2 weekly sessions are advised for a total of 6 to 8 sessions. A meta-analysis of 11 clinical trials, of which 5 are randomized clinical trials, concluded that ESWT improves the degree of cellulite. However, long-term follow-up data beyond 1 year are lacking.[33]

Radiofrequency

Radiofrequency (RF) waves are used to heat the dermis and subcutaneous tissue, thus inducing dermal remodeling, localized lipolysis, and improved microcirculation. Limitations of radiofrequency include short-lived results and the need for several sessions. There are several types of RF devices, and they vary depending on the electrode configuration (unipolar, monopolar, bipolar, tripolar, multipolar) and the combination with other technologies such as vacuum suction, laser/light, or pulsed electromagnetic fields. Many RF devices have been approved by the FDA for temporary reduction in the appearance of cellulite such as VelaSmooth and Velashape, which combine near-infrared light, bipolar radiofrequency, and mechanical suction; Venus Legacy, a multipolar RF device with pulsed magnetic fields; and Exilis Elite, which uses ultrasound and monopolar radiofrequency, among others.[34]

A study evaluated the efficacy of 8 weekly treatments with Venus Legacy for the treatment of abdominal cellulite in 25 healthy women. A reduction in subcutaneous thickness was observed at 1 week after treatment initiation, and improvement was noted by patients and a blinded investigator. Results were maintained 12 weeks after the completion of the treatment protocol.[35] In a study by Sadick and Magro, 16 women with cellulite on the thighs and/or buttocks were treated twice weekly for 6 weeks with VelaSmooth. The overall thigh circumference decreased in 71.87% of the treated legs. There was significant visual improvement in cellulite and skin texture.[36]

Subcision

The goal of subcision is to break the connective tissue septae, leading to a better redistribution of tension and fat lobules, and to induce controlled tissue injury, resulting in collagen stimulation. It is recommended only for cellulite depressions present at rest and not for those that are only apparent on muscle contraction. Subcision may be manual, vacuum-assisted, or laser-assisted. Manual subcision is performed with a needle or cannula. First, the area to be treated and depressions are marked with the patient in a standing position. Percutaneous infiltration of dilute lidocaine with epinephrine is then performed; this helps to anesthetize the area, achieve hemostasis, and separate the subcutaneous tissue from underlying structures. After 15 minutes, a forked cannula or an 18-G noncoring needle is inserted into the subcutaneous adipose tissue layer, parallel to the skin surface, at a depth of 10 to 20 mm. After the procedure, compression is recommended for 5 to 10 minutes to control bleeding. The main side effects include discomfort, pain, edema, bruising, and hemosiderosis.[23]

In a retrospective study, 232 women underwent manual subcision, with a 78.87% satisfaction rate after a single treatment session. Twenty-three patients were followed-up 2 years after the procedure with persistent results. An excessive response characterized by elevation of the treated area was observed in 14.22% of patients. The investigators attributed this response to 2 factors: (1) excessive surgical trauma resulting in excessive inflammation and collagen stimulation and (2) subcision done too superficially leading to the separation of the upper layer of subcutaneous fat from the lower layers. In cases of an excessive healing response, intralesional corticosteroids were effective in improving tissue elevation.[37]

Given the technique dependence of manual subcision, a vacuum-assisted system (Cellfina) was developed and FDA-approved for the treatment of cellulite. It allows users to select the exact depth of penetration and area of treatment. The vacuum-assisted design has a 0.45-mm microblade that can move forward and backward as well as side to side.[38] In 3 multicenter studies, a single treatment session of vacuum-assisted precise tissue release was safe and effective for the treatment of cellulite.[38–40]

Two recent multicenter studies evaluated the safety and efficacy of a new device for targeted verifiable subcision to reduce the appearance of moderate-to-severe cellulite in adult women. The device (now known as Avéli) is advanced through a small skin entry site. The distal end has a light to be able to track the location and depth and a hook to release the fibrous septae. The device was highly effective in reducing cellulite on the buttocks and thighs of adult women having an average of 20 depressions. Adverse events were mostly mild and expected for this type of procedure.[41,42]

Laser energy can also be used to break down the fibrous septae, induce local lipolysis, and stimulate collagen remodeling. The main device used for cellulite is a 1440 nm laser with a side-firing fiber tip (Cellulaze). In a prospective study of 25 women with grade II to III thigh cellulite, 1000 to 1500J of laser energy was delivered to treatment areas. Blinded evaluators and study subjects noted improvement after a single treatment session. Furthermore, objective measurement tools demonstrated an increase in mean skin elasticity and mean dermal thickness maintained 2 years after treatment.[43] In 2 other studies of women with buttock and thigh cellulite, improvement was noted by blinded investigators and was maintained at 6-month[44] and 1-year[45] follow-up.

Collagenase Clostridium Histolyticum

Collagenase enzymes isolated and purified from the fermentation of Clostridium histolyticum were approved by the FDA in 2020 for the treatment of moderate-to-severe cellulite in the buttocks of adult women. A different formulation of these enzymes is FDA-approved for the treatment of collagen-associated disorders (Peyronie disease and Dupytren contracture).

Collagenase Clostridium histolyticum-aaes (CCH-aaes; Qwo) is composed of 2 classes of collagenases known as AUX-I and AUX-II, mixed in a 1:1 ratio. These enzymes hydrolyze type I and III collagen, resulting in disruption of the fibrous septae in cellulite. The mechanism of action is enzymatic subcision and remodeling. CCH-aaes acts locally, and there is no systemic absorption.[46,47]

Two phase 2 and two phase 3 studies have demonstrated the efficacy of CCH-aaes for improving the appearance of cellulite on the buttocks.[46,48,49] A pooled analysis of 2 phase 3 trials

(RELEASE-1 and RELEASE-2) was conducted. A total of 843 women with moderate-to-severe cellulite on the buttocks were included, with 89.6% completing the studies. Four hundred twenty-four women received CCH-aaes injections, and 419 received placebo for up to 3 treatment sessions (days 1, 22, and 43). Twelve dimples were treated per patient with a total dose of 0.84 mg of CCH-aaes. Each injection dose (0.07 mg of CCH-aaes 0.23 mg/mL or placebo) was delivered as an injection of 3 0.1 mL aliquots. The initial aliquot was administered with the needle perpendicular to the skin surface. For the second and third aliquots, the needle was withdrawn slightly and oriented 45° toward the head and 45° toward the feet off the perpendicular axis. Subgroup analysis showed higher response rates in those with a lower age and body mass index less than 32 kg/m^2. Patient selection might therefore be essential for optimal results. The most common adverse events were pain, bruising, and injection-site nodule.[47]

A study evaluated 5 injection techniques of CCH-aaes in 63 women with buttock or thigh cellulite: technique A = shallow injection/3 aliquots; technique B = shallow injection/1 aliquot; technique C = deep injection/1 aliquot; technique D = deep and shallow injections/5 aliquots; or technique E = shallow injection/4 aliquots. For buttock cellulite, technique A resulted in the greatest improvement in CSS score on day 71. For thigh cellulite, CSS score improvement was greatest with technique D.[50]

Collagen Biostimulators

Calcium hydroxyapatite (CaHA) and poly-L-lactic acid (PLLA) are the most commonly used biostimulatory agents for skin tightening and lifting in the buttocks and thighs. Although these agents have shown great promise for the treatment of cellulite, further well-designed studies are needed to establish their efficacy and safety.

Radiesse contains CaHA microspheres suspended in a sodium carboxymethylcellulose gel carrier. When used undiluted or slightly diluted, it provides immediate volume correction (due to the carrier gel) that is gradually followed by collagen stimulation and new tissue formation. When used in a hyperdiluted form (ie, 1.5 mL of product plus ≥1.5 mL of diluent), Radiesse does not have a significant volumizing effect but it rather stimulates long-term tissue remodeling. In recent years, it has been increasingly used in a hyperdiluted form as a biostimulatory agent to improve skin quality and firmness on the face and body. An expert consensus provides guidance for the use of CaHA as a biostimulatory agent for face and body

rejuvenation. To improve skin laxity in the buttocks and thighs and reduce cellulite, the product should be injected mainly in the upper and lateral portions of the buttocks, the inner and posterior thigh areas, and in cellulite dimples. Usually, 1 syringe per buttock side or per thigh area (inner or posterior) is indicated per session. For buttocks and thigh skin laxity, the dilution may range from 1:1 to 1:4 (1.5–6 mL of diluent), whereas for cellulite dimples, lower dilutions (1:1 or 1:2) may be used.[51] Another global panel of experts defines hyperdiluted CaHA as CaHA reconstituted using ratios of 1:2 or higher (ie, 1.5 mL of product plus ≥3 mL of diluent). For cellulite, panel members recommend CaHA diluted 1:1 with lidocaine injected subdermally using a vectored-fanning approach. One to three sessions are required during the first year to achieve optimal results, with maintenance injections every 12 to 18 months thereafter.[52] The combination of diluted CaHA injected immediately after the use of Microfocused Ultrasound with Visualization has been shown to significantly improve the appearance of cellulite.[53]

PLLA is another popular biostimulatory agent. It induces an inflammatory tissue response whereby the injected microparticles are encapsulated by host immune cells, leading to neocollagenesis and increased dermal thickness.[54]

An expert consensus provides guidance for the use of PLLA for contour deficiencies of the buttocks. The product can be used immediately after reconstitution. It may also be reconstituted up to 3 days before injection. A larger amount of product is usually needed for volumization than for textural irregularities, but typically at least 1 to 2 vials per side of the buttocks per session are needed. Up to 3 treatment sessions are recommended, 4 to 6 weeks apart. PLLA is reconstituted with sterile or bacteriostatic water before use. The recommended volume for injection is 18 mL, including an optional 1 mL of 1% lidocaine. To address textural changes and cellulite, the injection plane should be the superficial fat layer. For volume enhancement, deep injections should be administered in the upper outer quadrant of the buttocks only, as this quadrant is the safest for injection in this layer. Injections should be superficial in the other quadrants.[55]

Two studies by Mazzuco and colleagues showed the efficacy of PLLA injections with[56] and without[57] subcision for the treatment of cellulite and for gluteal augmentation and contouring. PLLA was diluted in 10 mL of sterile water for injection, 48 to 96 hours before the procedure. At the time of the injections, 2 mL of 2% lidocaine was added to the PLLA preparation, and the injections were done using a needle or cannula. Two to four vials were used per session, and 1 to 4 treatment sessions were done. In another randomized, double-blind, placebo-controlled study, repeated PLLA treatments combined with subcision were effective and safe in improving the appearance of cellulite.[58]

CLINICS CARE POINTS

- Cellulite affects around 85% to 98% of post-pubertal women.
- Physicians should make their patients aware of the unpredictable efficacy of treatment and the potential for only short-term improvement despite several treatment sessions.
- Combining different therapeutic modalities is advised for better and longer-lasting results.

FUNDING SOURCES

None.

CONFLICTS OF INTEREST

None declared.

ACKNOWLEDGMENTS

The authors would like to thank Mrs Cosette Khalil for the illustration (see **Fig. 1**).

REFERENCES

1. Avram MM. Cellulite: a review of its physiology and treatment. J Cosmet Laser Ther 2004;6(4):181–5.
2. Davis DS, Boen M, Fabi SG. Cellulite: patient selection and combination treatments for optimal results—a review and our experience. Dermatol Surg 2019;45(9):1171–84.
3. Arora G, Patil A, Hooshanginezhad Z, et al. Cellulite: Presentation and management. J Cosmet Dermatol 2022;21(4):1393–401.
4. Hexsel D, Siega C, Schilling-Souza J, et al. Assessment of psychological, psychiatric, and behavioral aspects of patients with cellulite: a pilot study. Surg Cosmet Dermatol 2012;4(2):131–6.
5. Rossi AM, Katz BE. A modern approach to the treatment of cellulite. Dermatol Clin 2014;32(1):51–9.
6. Hexsel D, Valente Bezerra I, Mosena G, et al. Considerations on zero-degree cellulite. J Cosmet Dermatol 2022;21(1):134–6.
7. Nurnberger F, Muller G. So-called cellulite: an invented disease. J Dermatol Surg Oncol 1978;4(3):221–9.
8. Rudolph C, Hladik C, Hamade H, et al. Structural Gender Dimorphism and the Biomechanics of the Gluteal Subcutaneous Tissue: Implications for the Pathophysiology of Cellulite. Plast Reconstr Surg 2019;143(4):1077–86.
9. Querleux B, Cornillon C, Jolivet O, et al. Anatomy and physiology of subcutaneous adipose tissue by in vivo magnetic resonance imaging and spectroscopy: relationships with sex and presence of cellulite. Skin Res Technol 2002;8(2):118–24.
10. Mirrashed F, Sharp JC, Krause V, et al. Pilot study of dermal and subcutaneous fat structures by MRI in individuals who differ in gender, BMI, and cellulite grading. Skin Res Technol 2004;10(3):161–8.
11. Pierard GE, Nizet JL, Pierard-Franchimont C. Cellulite: from standing fat herniation to hypodermal stretch marks. Am J Dermatopathol 2000;22(1):34–7.
12. Hexsel DM, Abreu M, Rodrigues TC, et al. Side-by-side comparison of areas with and without cellulite depressions using magnetic resonance imaging. Dermatol Surg 2009;35(10):1471–7.
13. Curri S, Bombardelli E. Local lipodystrophy and districtual microcirculation. Cosmet Toilet 1994;109(9):51–65.
14. Lotti T, Ghersetich I, Grappone C, et al. Proteoglycans in so-called cellulite. Int J Dermatol 1990;29(4):272–4.
15. Rosenbaum M, Prieto V, Hellmer J, et al. An exploratory investigation of the morphology and biochemistry of cellulite. Plast Reconstr Surg 1998;101(7):1934–9.
16. Tokarska K, Tokarski S, Wozniacka A, et al. Cellulite: a cosmetic or systemic issue? Contemporary views on the etiopathogenesis of cellulite. Postepy Dermatol Alergol 2018;35(5):442–6.
17. Philip K, Blackburn MR. The hypoxic adenosine response and inflammation in Lung disease. Academic Press: Translational Inflammation: Elsevier; 2019. p. 23–41.
18. Emanuele E, Bertona M, Geroldi D. A multilocus candidate approach identifies ACE and HIF1A as susceptibility genes for cellulite. J Eur Acad Dermatol Venereol 2010;24(8):930–5.
19. Tomczyk M, Nowak W, Jaźwa A. Endothelium in physiology and pathogenesis of diseases. Postepy Biochem 2013;59(4):357–64.
20. Kligman A. Cellulite: facts and fiction. J Geriatr Dermatol 1997;5(4):136–9.
21. Scherwitz C, Braun-Falco O. So-called cellulite. J Dermatol Surg Oncol 1978;4(3):230–4.
22. Bass LS, Kaminer MS. Insights Into the Pathophysiology of Cellulite: A Review. Dermatol Surg 2020;46(Suppl 1):S77–85.
23. Friedmann DP, Vick GL, Mishra V. Cellulite: a review with a focus on subcision. Clin Cosmet Investig Dermatol 2017;10:17–23.
24. Hexsel DM, Dal'forno T, Hexsel CL. A validated photonumeric cellulite severity scale. J Eur Acad Dermatol Venereol 2009;23(5):523–8.

25. Hexsel D, Fabi SG, Sattler G, et al. Validated Assessment Scales for Cellulite Dimples on the Buttocks and Thighs in Female Patients. Dermatol Surg 2019;45(Suppl 1):S2–11.

26. Young VL, DiBernardo BE. Comparison of Cellulite Severity Scales and Imaging Methods. Aesthetic Surg J 2021;41(6):NP521–37.

27. Rossi AB, Vergnanini AL. Cellulite: a review. J Eur Acad Dermatol Venereol 2000;14(4):251–62.

28. Taati B, Khoshnoodnasab M. Exercise-based approaches to the treatment of cellulite. International Journal of Medical Reviews 2019;6(1):26–7.

29. Smalls LK, Hicks M, Passeretti D, et al. Effect of weight loss on cellulite: gynoid lypodystrophy. Plast Reconstr Surg 2006;118(2):510–6.

30. Turati F, Pelucchi C, Marzatico F, et al. Efficacy of cosmetic products in cellulite reduction: systematic review and meta-analysis. J Eur Acad Dermatol Venereol 2014;28(1):1–15.

31. Gulec AT. Treatment of cellulite with LPG endermologie. Int J Dermatol 2009;48(3):265–70.

32. Kutlubay Z, Songur A, Engsmall i UB, et al. An alternative treatment modality for cellulite: LPG endermologie. J Cosmet Laser Ther 2013;15(5):266–70.

33. Knobloch K, Kraemer R. Extracorporeal shock wave therapy (ESWT) for the treatment of cellulite–A current metaanalysis. Int J Surg 2015;24(Pt B):210–7.

34. Ferzli G, Sadick N. A review of current modalities to treat cellulite effectively. Dermatological Reviews 2020;1(4):123–7.

35. Wanitphakdeedecha R, Sathaworawong A, Manuskiatti W, et al. Efficacy of multipolar radiofrequency with pulsed magnetic field therapy for the treatment of abdominal cellulite. J Cosmet Laser Ther 2017;19(4):205–9.

36. Sadick N, Magro C. A study evaluating the safety and efficacy of the VelaSmooth system in the treatment of cellulite. J Cosmet Laser Ther 2007;9(1):15–20.

37. Hexsel DM, Mazzuco R. Subcision: a treatment for cellulite. Int J Dermatol 2000;39(7):539–44.

38. Kaminer MS, Coleman WP 3rd, Weiss RA, et al. A Multicenter Pivotal Study to Evaluate Tissue Stabilized-Guided Subcision Using the Cellfina Device for the Treatment of Cellulite With 3-Year Follow-Up. Dermatol Surg 2017;43(10):1240–8.

39. Kaminer MS, Coleman WP 3rd, Weiss RA, et al. Multicenter pivotal study of vacuum-assisted precise tissue release for the treatment of cellulite. Dermatol Surg 2015;41(3):336–47.

40. Guida S, Bovani B, Canta Pier L, et al. Multicenter study of vacuum-assisted precise tissue release for the treatment of cellulite in a cohort of 112 Italian women assessed with cellulite dimples scale at rest. J Cosmet Laser Ther 2019;21(7–8):404–7.

41. Stevens WG, Green JB, Layt C, et al. Multicenter Pivotal Study Demonstrates Safety and Efficacy of a New Cellulite Procedure: Final Results at 12 Months. Aesthetic Surg J 2022;43(1):97–108.

42. Stevens WG, Kaminer MS, Fabi SG, et al. Study of a New Controlled Focal Septa Release Cellulite Reduction Method. Aesthetic Surg J 2022;42(8):937–45.

43. Sasaki GH. Single treatment of grades II and III cellulite using a minimally invasive 1,440-nm pulsed Nd:YAG laser and side-firing fiber: an institutional review board-approved study with a 24-month follow-up period. Aesthetic Plast Surg 2013;37:1073–89.

44. Katz B. Quantitative & qualitative evaluation of the efficacy of a 1440 nm Nd: YAG laser with novel bidirectional optical fiber in the treatment of cellulite as measured by 3-dimensional surface imaging. J Drugs Dermatol JDD 2013;12(11):1224–30.

45. DiBernardo BE, Sasaki GH, Katz BE, et al. A Multicenter Study for Cellulite Treatment Using a 1440-nm Nd:YAG Wavelength Laser with Side-Firing Fiber. Aesthetic Surg J 2016;36(3):335–43.

46. Sadick NS, Goldman MP, Liu G, et al. Collagenase Clostridium Histolyticum for the Treatment of Edematous Fibrosclerotic Panniculopathy (Cellulite): A Randomized Trial. Dermatol Surg 2019;45(8):1047–56.

47. Bass LS, Kaufman-Janette J, Joseph JH, et al. Collagenase Clostridium Histolyticum-aaes for Treatment of Cellulite: A Pooled Analysis of Two Phase-3 Trials. Plast Reconstr Surg Glob Open 2022;10(5):e4306.

48. Kaufman-Janette J, Joseph JH, Kaminer MS, et al. Collagenase Clostridium Histolyticum-aaes for the Treatment of Cellulite in Women: Results From Two Phase 3 Randomized, Placebo-Controlled Trials. Dermatol Surg 2021;47(5):649–56.

49. Kaufman-Janette JA, Bass LS, Xiang Q, et al. Efficacy, Safety, and Durability of Response of Collagenase Clostridium Histolyticum-aaes for Treating Cellulite. Plast Reconstr Surg Glob Open 2020;8(12):e3316.

50. Kaufman-Janette J, Katz BE, Vijayan S, et al. Evaluation of five collagenase clostridium histolyticum-aaes injection techniques for the treatment of cellulite on the buttock or thigh. J Cosmet Dermatol 2022;21(4):1448–53.

51. de Almeida AT, Figueredo V, da Cunha ALG, et al. Consensus recommendations for the use of hyperdiluted calcium hydroxyapatite (Radiesse) as a face and body biostimulatory agent. Plastic and Reconstructive Surgery Global Open 2019;7(3).

52. Goldie K, Peeters W, Alghoul M, et al. Global consensus guidelines for the injection of diluted and hyperdiluted calcium hydroxylapatite for skin tightening. Dermatol Surg 2018;44:S32–41.

53. Casabona G, Pereira G. Microfocused Ultrasound with Visualization and Calcium Hydroxylapatite for Improving Skin Laxity and Cellulite Appearance. Plast Reconstr Surg Glob Open 2017;5(7):e1388.

54. Christen M-O. Collagen stimulators in body applications: a review focused on poly-L-lactic acid (PLLA). Clin Cosmet Invest Dermatol 2022:997–1019.

55. Harper J, Avelar L, Haddad A, et al. Expert Recommendations on the Use of Injectable Poly-L-lactic Acid for Contour Deficiencies of the Buttocks. J Drugs Dermatol JDD 2022;21(1):21–6.
56. Mazzuco R. Subcision plus poly-l-lactic acid for the treatment of cellulite associated to flaccidity in the buttocks and thighs. J Cosmet Dermatol 2020; 19(5):1165–71.
57. Mazzuco R, Dal'Forno T, Hexsel D. Poly-L-Lactic Acid for Nonfacial Skin Laxity. Dermatol Surg 2020; 46(Suppl 1):S86–8.
58. Swearingen A, Medrano K, Ferzli G, et al. Randomized, Double-Blind, Placebo-Controlled Study of Poly-L-Lactic acid for Treatment of Cellulite in the Lower Extremities. J Drugs Dermatol 2021;20(5): 529–33.